RESTORING
FISCAL SANITY
——— 2007 ———

ALICE M. RIVLIN *and* JOSEPH R. ANTOS
Editors

RESTORING
FISCAL SANITY
—— 2007 ——

The Health Spending Challenge

BROOKINGS INSTITUTION PRESS
Washington, D.C.

Copyright © 2007
THE BROOKINGS INSTITUTION
1775 Massachusetts Avenue, N.W., Washington, D.C. 20036
www.brookings.edu

Library of Congress Cataloging-in-Publication data

Restoring fiscal sanity 2007 : the health spending challenge / Alice M. Rivlin and Joseph R. Antos, editors.
   p. ; cm.
Includes bibliographical references and index.
Summary: "Authors suggest reforms in federal programs that have the potential to reduce the growth of spending for the entire health system, increase the efficiency and effectiveness of care provided, and enhance health outcomes and stress the need for innovative approaches and cooperation between the private and public sectors"—Provided by publisher.
   ISBN-13: 978-0-8157-7493-8 (pbk. : alk. paper)
   ISBN-10: 0-8157-7493-1 (pbk. : alk. paper)
   1. Medical care, Cost of—United States. 2. Medical care—United States—Cost control. 3. Health care reform—Economic aspects—United States. 4. Medical economics—United States. I. Rivlin, Alice M. II. Antos, Joseph R. III. Brookings Institution.
   [DNLM: 1. Health Expenditures—United States. 2. Health Care Reform—economics—United States. 3. National Health Programs—economics—United States. W 74 AA1 R398 2007]

RA410.53.R488 2007
362.1'0425—dc22   2007000586

1 3 5 7 9 8 6 4 2

Typeset in Sabon

Composition by Cynthia Stock
Silver Spring, Maryland

Printed by Victor Graphics
Baltimore, Maryland

Contents

Foreword   vii

Acknowledgments   xi

Overview   1

1   Rising Health Care Spending—Federal and National   13
    Joseph R. Antos and Alice M. Rivlin

2   Strategies for Slowing the Growth of Health Spending   29
    Joseph R. Antos and Alice M. Rivlin

3   The Challenge of Medicare   81
    Gail R. Wilensky

4   The Role of Medicaid   105
    Alan R. Weil and Louis F. Rossiter

5   Leveraging Other Federal Health Systems   131
    Susan D. Hosek

6   Private Payer Roles in Moving to More Efficient
    Health Spending   153
    Paul B. Ginsburg

7 Cost Containment and the Politics of Health Care Reform 173
Judith Feder and Donald W. Moran

8 Building Public Support for Slowing the Growth
of Health Care Spending 193
Stuart M. Butler

Contributors 219
Index 221

Foreword

Our ongoing search for ways to restore fiscal sanity to the federal budget is a Brookings project that does the Institution proud. It meets the highest standards of quality research and constructive policy prescriptions. This volume, the third in the series, could not be timelier: first, because health care reform is very much on the minds of Americans and their elected leaders and, second, because it is particularly on our minds at Brookings. We are going to be making the subject a priority for at least the next decade.

While there are many dimensions to the issue, economics is at its core. Health care spending in the United States now exceeds $2 trillion annually—close to 17 percent of all spending—and is growing significantly faster than the national economy. If health spending continues to grow at historical rates it will threaten the ability of many Americans to pay for other essential services. It is important to be sure that we are getting our money's worth for this huge expenditure. Federal government health expenditures—driven primarily by promises to a growing senior population under Medicare and Medicaid—are a rapidly ballooning share of the federal budget and are projected to grow considerably faster than federal revenues at current tax rates. Unless the growth of federal health spending can be slowed, Americans will face difficult choices involving paying substantially higher taxes, making sharp reductions in other government programs, and reneging on promises to the elderly.

This book is designed to focus attention on an urgent problem and help citizens evaluate a wide range of approaches to slowing the growth of spending on health care. Acknowledging the complexity of the problem, Joseph Antos and Alice Rivlin, the editors of this volume, reject the idea that there is one silver bullet solution—or even a handful. Recognizing that rising health care spending is a problem that reaches beyond the federal government, the authors avoid policies that simply shift costs to the states or the private sector. Instead, they focus on reforms in federal programs that have the potential to reduce the growth of spending for the entire health system, increase the efficiency and effectiveness of the care provided, and enhance health outcomes.

A word about the editors: Alice Rivlin, a senior fellow in our Economic Studies program, is something of an institution herself—and, I can add on the basis of my own experience, an exemplary colleague. I have had the honor of working with her both at Brookings and before that in government. She was the founding director of the Congressional Budget Office and served as director of the Office of Management and Budget in the Clinton administration. Joseph Antos is a health economist at the American Enterprise Institute, our neighbor and frequent partner. He, too, has served at the Congressional Budget Office.

Alice and Joe have assembled a diverse group of policy experts whose views and experience span the political spectrum. Several have served in senior positions in Republican and Democratic administrations. As a group, they have had hands-on experience in Congress, the executive branch of the federal government, state governments, and the private sector. Although these experts write from varying perspectives and hold different opinions on the best approaches to reform, they all stress the need for innovative approaches and cooperation between the private and public sectors. They have a shared view of the importance of reforming federal health programs in ways that not only reduce future federal budget deficits but also move the whole health system toward higher quality, greater efficiency, broader coverage, and slower overall health spending growth.

Their work, as assembled here, is an important contribution to intelligent debate and the search for bold but practical solutions to one of the biggest challenges facing our nation.

STROBE TALBOTT
President

Washington, D.C.
January 2007

Acknowledgments

Brookings is grateful to the Annie E. Casey Foundation, the Charles Stewart Mott Foundation, and the Harry and Jeanette Weinberg Foundation for their continuing support of this project, but acknowledges that the findings and conclusions presented here are those of the authors alone and do not necessarily reflect the opinions of the foundations.

For their advice and support, we thank the members of the corporate advisory committee for the Budgeting for National Priorities project. Formed under the leadership of Geoffrey Boisi, the committee includes Raymond Chambers, Richard Dumler, Fred Gluck, Thomas Healey, Robert Kaplan, Edward M. Lamont, Jr., Robert Marks, Thomas Saunders III, and Roy Zuckerberg.

The editors are extremely grateful to all the authors—Stuart Butler, Judith Feder, Paul Ginsburg, Susan Hosek, Donald Moran, Louis Rossiter, Alan Weil, and Gail Wilensky—for working so hard on this project, despite their many other commitments, and contributing so much. The dialogue at the authors' conference, as well as ongoing feedback throughout the writing and editing process, helped create a thoughtful, coherent volume on a very complex subject.

Isabel Sawhill provided helpful advice and strong support for the project at all stages. We are also grateful for insightful comments from William Gale, James Capretta, and two anonymous reviewers.

Special thanks are due to Porsha Cropper and Marni Schultz for their expert research assistance; Marty Gottron and Anthony Nathe for editing; Anne Hardenbergh and Andrea Kane for outreach; Sabrina Fisher, Eric Haven, and Emily Roessel for research verification; Larry Converse for typesetting and printing; Susan Woollen for cover design coordination; Julia Petrakis for indexing; Inge Lockwood for proofreading; Evelyn Taylor for administrative assistance; and Marni Schultz for coordinating the editing and production processes.

Overview

Over the past half century, most Americans have experienced increased prosperity and improved quality of life. We are living longer, and advances in knowledge and technology have made medical care increasingly effective and are likely to continue to do so. But these triumphs pose serious challenges. As health care improves, Americans are spending higher proportions of their income to obtain it. Health care is crowding out other spending by individuals, businesses, and government. Moreover, our complex, fragmented health care system is demonstrably inefficient and unnecessarily costly. Americans are increasingly concerned that they are spending a great deal on medical care and not getting their money's worth. The rising cost of care is making health care coverage less affordable and adding to the already substantial ranks of the uninsured.

The health spending challenge shows up strikingly in the federal budget, where the cost of federal health programs, primarily health care promises to the elderly, is projected to grow substantially faster than federal revenues at current tax rates. The projected growth of federal health spending will force tough decisions about the federal budget. If past trends in health care spending continue it will not be possible to keep promises made to the elderly and other vulnerable populations without large continuous tax increases, even if other federal spending is drastically curtailed. Indeed, if current programs remain in place and recent health spending trends continue, within a generation the cost of Medicare and Medicaid alone will exceed the amount of national resources historically devoted to financing the whole federal government. This rapid projected growth is partly attributable to demographics—the retirement of the large baby-boom generation and the fact that Americans are living longer. More important, it is due to the fact that Americans are consuming more and increasingly expensive health care, whether that care is financed by the government or the private sector. Health care spending dominates the future federal budget crunch. If health care could be delivered more efficiently, federal budget choices would be far less agonizing.

But federal health programs are only pieces of a larger picture. Health spending is putting pressure on the budgets of families, businesses, non-profit enterprises, states, and communities. Total national spending for health care—now approaching 17 percent of all spending—continues to rise rapidly. Attempts to reduce federal spending by cutting Medicare and Medicaid benefits and restricting eligibility will only serve to shift the burden to other payers without reforming the system in ways that could improve the effectiveness of health care or slow the growth of total spending.

Although Americans devote a considerably higher proportion of total resources to health care than people in other advanced countries, their health outcomes are worse, millions remain without health insurance, and there is considerable evidence that the health care delivery system is inefficient and wasteful. The size of the federal health programs makes their leadership essential to systemic reform. The challenging question addressed in this book is: how can federal health care programs be reformed in ways that slow the growth of total health spending and move the whole system toward greater efficiency and effectiveness, broader coverage, and better health outcomes?

Rising Health Care Spending—Federal and National

In chapter 1 we focus on current projections of health care spending. We discuss why health care spending is rising so rapidly in the United States and other developed countries. We show the dramatic effect that current rates of growth in health care programs will have on the federal budget and why we believe such growth to be unsustainable.

Strategies for Slowing the Growth of Health Spending

In chapter 2 we assess a broad range of options that could slow spending or improve long-term performance of federal health programs, while taking into consideration the interconnectedness of the entire health system. Previous attempts to reform federal health programs have often been myopic, taking aim at short-term budget scores rather than long-term efficiency; these approaches often succeed only in shifting costs to the private sector, rather than reducing total health spending.

Comprehensive reform of the U.S. health system will eventually be necessary if we are to achieve efficient production of effective, high-value health care with a rate of spending growth that can be sustained well into the future. Most policy proposals to reduce growth in health spending take one of two approaches to reform—market based or regulatory based. Market strategies rely on informed consumers who respond to greater competition by making cost-effective choices that will improve quality of care and lower costs. Regulatory strategies, by contrast, promote active government intervention through administrative rules on reimbursement rates, provider performance, or total spending to achieve the same ends.

Whether reform should move toward universal health care under a single-payer system or greater competition among private health plans has long been debated by experts, including many of the authors of this volume. We argue in chapter 2 that the country should not wait to resolve the conceptual debate over health reform before taking actions that can squeeze out inefficiency and promote better functioning of federal health programs and the health system at large. The problems are both large and complex, and solutions will inevitably involve a blend of regulatory and market elements. Consequently, many different approaches should be tried to improve efficiency, to slow health spending growth, and to promote a more equitable system. Improved information about treatment effectiveness, costs, and outcomes is critical to any strategy pursued.

Some policy proposals—such as health information technology, disease prevention, malpractice reform, and pay-for-performance—have been touted as the keys to better health care at lower cost for everyone. Unfortunately, there are no silver bullets. Although those proposals have considerable merit, no single proposal can solve the entire spending problem by itself, and each proposal requires a considerable investment of money and effort to become effective. Such ideas should be part of a broader agenda of experimentation and reform.

Many policy options considered in this chapter are likely to yield one-time savings rather than a permanent reduction in the growth of federal health outlays. Although perhaps not ideal, at least adopting such an approach would buy time for further policy development and innovation. We argue that there is no lack of policy ideas to test, but there may be a lack of political will to proceed.

Broader health system reform is not possible without implementing changes in federal programs and health-related activities. Medicare and Medicaid account for such a large share of total health spending that they must be part of wider efforts to improve health care. Federal tax subsidies help millions of workers purchase private insurance through their employers, but those subsidies could be revamped to better target those in need and minimize incentives that promote inefficient use of health services. Regulatory agencies, including the Federal Trade Commission and the Food and Drug Administration, establish the legal framework for competition in the health sector and provide important consumer protections.

Federal leadership can provide a catalyst for developing and implementing significant reforms by public and private insurers and health plans. Medicare is testing ways to improve payment and delivery systems that could increase the quality of care and reduce program spending. Many states have undertaken projects to improve the operation of their Medicaid programs. The Veterans Health Administration has led the way in developing electronic medical records and improving communications within the VA health system. Lessons from these efforts can be adopted by other health programs, both public and private.

The challenge of rising health care spending will not be resolved in the near term; at best, it will be mitigated and managed through many small but significant steps. Ultimately, Americans will be forced to decide how much of their individual and national resources to allocate to extending life and how increasingly expensive care will be allocated among citizens. A large number of reforms must be implemented over an extended period of time if we are to reduce growth in health spending while enhancing the effectiveness of care. Although some proposals in this book may preclude others, we believe that many can and should be pursued simultaneously.

The Challenge of Medicare

In chapter 3 Gail Wilensky emphasizes the interconnectedness of efforts to slow spending growth in Medicare and in the health system as a whole. The size of the Medicare program, coupled with the political unlikelihood that Medicare spending growth will be allowed to fall behind growth in total health care spending, means that future Medicare spending growth will help signal the success or failure of efforts to moderate spending growth across the system.

Medicare is currently undertaking several demonstration programs to change provider incentives in ways that will reward quality and encourage efficiency. If these prove successful, they could hold tremendous value for both Medicare and private health insurers. Political realities—a growing senior population that is unlikely to tolerate differences between Medicare and the private sector regarding access to new technologies or high-priced providers—suggest that Medicare and private-sector spending streams are likely to converge over time. Thus sustaining efficiency and lower spending growth in one system will occur only if there are comparable changes in the other system.

Wilensky reviews a range of proposals to slow spending in the Medicare program, including constraining provider payments and increasing the eligibility age and cost sharing by beneficiaries, and weighs the political likelihood and financial impacts of each. Similar to other authors in this volume, she sees the most promise for moderating spending in promoting efficient, high-quality care. Specifically, she recommends development of a national performance measurement system that would use comparative clinical effectiveness information to reward providers for high-quality, appropriate care. Investing in such a system would be an important role for the federal government—one that would realign financial incentives and enable improved care throughout the health system.

The Role of Medicaid

While Medicaid represents a significantly smaller share of the federal budget than Medicare, its anticipated rate of growth is slightly higher than that of Medicare and substantially more than anticipated growth in federal revenues. In chapter 4 Alan Weil and Louis Rossiter explore a variety of approaches that could control Medicaid's rate of growth. They note that Medicaid was established out of recognition that low-income Americans could not adequately access the health care system—any attempts to cut costs by reducing covered services or program eligibility risk recreating those problems. Instead, they believe cost solutions must be found through greater efficiency and consider several policy levers to accomplish this.

To change the incentives that states face in making Medicaid policy decisions, Weil and Rossiter consider the consequences of converting Medicaid into a block grant to states. They conclude that, while this would certainly help control federal Medicaid spending, such an approach would simply shift the financial risk to states and their beneficiaries. Another possibility is to design a generalized response to reduce the degree of fiscal gaming practiced by states. Medicaid costs could also be reduced by adopting reforms to change provider behavior, such as disease management, pay-for-performance, and managed care. These reforms are being used and showing promise in the private health sector. The authors also see possibility in a pair of policies designed to change the behavior of individual beneficiaries: Defined contributions allow beneficiaries to choose among plans that have the same costs but varying benefits, and financial incentives can encourage health-promoting behaviors, such as keeping doctor's appointments, adhering to drug treatment regimens, and lessening use of emergency rooms. Finally, they explore two ideas that could help reduce demand for Medicaid. One, establishing national eligibility standards based on financial need, would eliminate cross-state disparities and simplify program administration. The other, promoting private long-term care insurance through partnership programs, is still relatively untested but would likely remove some of the cost burden from both states and the federal government.

Leveraging Other Federal Health Systems

In chapter 5 Susan Hosek explores the growth of the Veterans Health Administration (VHA) and the Military Health System (MHS). Both systems face rising cost pressures resulting from the increasing attractiveness of their services relative to private health coverage. Over time the scope of benefits provided to veterans and military beneficiaries has grown, reaching a point today where these packages are significantly better than most private employer health plans. With these programs providing care that is of equal quality and lower cost, potential beneficiaries are increasingly switching out of private plans. Both the Department of Veterans Affairs and Department of Defense (DoD) have proposed modest increases in cost sharing to moderate the demand for care by current enrollees and to discourage additional eligible beneficiaries from shifting into these systems from private coverage. However, with so many military personnel deployed and at risk overseas, Congress has not supported these changes. One way to generate sizable cost savings for these programs is to update prescription co-pays to employer-plan levels, an approach that is less likely to encounter political resistance. VHA and MHS must also generate cost savings through improved efficiency.

VHA and MHS innovations—in efficiency and quality of care—could act as examples for the rest of the U.S. health sector. Development of electronic medical records (EMR) systems can improve care and save money. VHA pioneered the Veterans Health Information System and Technology Architecture (VistA), which it has made available to private-sector providers at nominal cost. DoD is close to full implementation of its EMR system, the Armed Forces Health Longitudinal Technology Application (AHLTA). Both systems can make valuable contributions to the entire health sector by sharing information on cost-effective design, implementation, and training requirements, as well as methods to exploit the systems to improve health outcomes. VHA has also become a leader in quality-of-care improvements, with its adoption of a quality improvement initiative that has resulted in higher standards of care by holding providers and managers accountable for measured quality performance. The federal government would be well served to encourage VHA and MHS to continue aggressively developing and testing new approaches to providing quality, lower-cost care, and disseminating this information to the broader health care sector.

Private Payer Roles in Moving to More Efficient Health Spending

In chapter 6 Paul Ginsburg emphasizes the links between the activities of private and public health insurers. He argues that not only will developments in private insurance have direct effects on the federal budget but that they will also have indirect effects by their influence on the degree to which reforms aimed directly at federal health programs can succeed. The exclusion from taxation of employer contributions to health insurance has an enormous effect on federal revenues, while direct subsidies for purchase of private insurance, especially for Medicare Part D prescription drug plans, represents another large federal health expense. Ginsburg highlights important indirect effects as well, which grow out of the reality that many providers treat patients with different kinds of health insurance coverage, both public and private. The result of this common delivery system is that strong initiatives from either payer—for instance, a change in payment policies to hospitals and physicians—will influence care across the board.

Given this interconnectedness, Ginsburg argues that tools to contain spending that are used in one sector can make the other sector more effective as well. Private payers are currently focused on the potential of patient financial incentives—higher co-payments, deductibles, and coinsurance—to reduce costs. These strategies could have an impact on federal health programs as well, especially their most successful feature—creating incentives for generic drug use. Another option, which better addresses the problem of concentrated expenses in a small number of enrollees, is the use of high-performance networks, where patients are directed toward high-performing physicians on the basis of quality and costs per episode of care. The federal government could spur development of this savings tool by providing data, such as access to Medicare claims, to create a larger sample for assessments of physician efficiency and quality. Pay-for-performance (P4P) is another potential incentive to promote higher quality care. For private insurers, the challenge is coordinating choice of measurements. Measures chosen by Medicare, which is currently conducting P4P demonstrations, would likely be agreed to by private insurers, thereby creating system-wide standards. The public and private health sectors should be open to adopting reform tools that reinforce cost-saving behavior across the entire system.

Cost Containment and the Politics of Health Care Reform

Reforming the health care system in this country has long been of interest to policymakers and citizens alike. However, despite much public debate, little of real substance has been accomplished. In chapter 7 Judith Feder and Donald Moran explore several major barriers to large-scale health reform and how they have played out recently in national politics. The Clinton administration's failed effort to implement reform faltered on a central reality of health care financing—unless policymakers are willing to spend more money, it is not possible to cover the uninsured without placing at least some restrictions on the already-insured. As the cost of existing care rises, it becomes increasingly difficult to expand coverage. First, rising costs create a larger uninsured population, as public and private insurance reduce coverage and some individuals opt out of these more limited options. Second, rising costs means greater subsidies are necessary for the uninsured to afford care, a redistributive situation that raises the political, as well as economic, costs of expanding coverage. The Clinton experience also demonstrated that even if new revenues can be identified to finance expanded coverage, the already-insured population will still be affected by whatever cost containment strategy is implemented to contain spending within this new health care budget.

Moving past the efforts during the Clinton era, health care reform continues to be debated in a highly charged environment. Beyond the generally perceived increase in polarization and interparty factionalism, the political environment holds particularly strong challenges for health care reformers. First, several of the hot button issues that engage and enrage ideological opposites fall within the health care realm, most notably abortion and stem cell research. Second, the fiscal importance of health spending as part of federal and state budgets has raised the stakes for reform efforts. Finally, the loss of moderates from the political scene strongly affects health care policy, as the size and complexity of the health care system require substantial legislative and regulatory action simply to ensure that the existing framework runs smoothly. As Feder and Moran note, the fractious efforts to implement the Medicare Modernization Act make it difficult "to visualize how to grow a political center large enough to take concerted action to restore fiscal sanity before the financial divide between promises and resources proves unbridgeable."

Building upon and validating the recommendations made in the preceding chapters, Feder and Moran conclude that the best hope for meaningful health reform lies with serious efforts to contain costs. In their opinion, this means recognizing that creation of a more economical health system will require many people to economize, and to do so efficiently will require policymakers to develop the evidence and processes to enable the system to rationally and acceptably say no. The generation of balanced, scientifically rigorous research to inform decisionmaking on coverage and reimbursement policies can help the public and private health systems to internalize incentives that promote cost-conscious care.

Building Public Support for Slowing the Growth of Health Care Spending

In chapter 8 Stuart Butler discusses the practical political considerations of transforming policy proposals into successful legislation. He observes that public opinion about health care policy is particularly complicated because people tend to view proposals in very personal and financial terms, as well as in terms of basic values. This volume discusses two approaches to spending control: improving the efficiency with which we spend health dollars and designing incentives or controls to limit expenditures. When addressing health care costs and spending, we are forced to consider obligations and responsibilities, how they are distributed in society, and who makes decisions. The market allows individuals choice, but it may not capture our social values.

Butler considers why our efforts focus on reducing health care costs, rather than simply improving efficiency in delivery of care. He identifies an important public policy reason for these efforts—health care spending is in competition with other policy goals and long-term promises made. Currently, the true costs of health spending are hidden from public consideration. Budget tradeoffs must be made more transparent and more public to assist difficult decisionmaking.

Butler raises a range of questions that force consideration of existing health obligations, and he sets forth possible paths in a cost-constrained future. He wonders what would happen if policymakers reconsidered the current promise of the Medicare social contract. Would Americans be willing to alter it to free up resources for other social goals? Perhaps we would tolerate transforming Medicare into income insurance that would protect an individual's ability to afford health care during retirement but that required higher-income retirees to pay a premium for coverage. As we work to balance the financial risks associated with health, decisions will have to be made on allocating resources. One approach is to allocate resources according to a community-wide sense of fairness and efficiency. Another supports investing control mainly with individual users of services and allowing the market to allocate resources in a manner that maximizes individual preferences. Butler argues that efforts to pursue policy refinements are more likely to succeed if proposals can be made more compatible with the underlying values of Americans—or at least proposed in ways that force the public to consider the moral trade-offs involved. Engaging citizens in serious discussions about these issues and values can strengthen efforts to generate strong public support for the necessary steps to rein in health care costs.

The rest of this book explores options for restoring fiscal sanity to our health care spending. By presenting a broad range of proposals, we hope to emphasize that solutions to this spending challenge are possible and that to have an impact the country needs to vigorously pursue a multi-pronged approach.

1

Rising Health Care Spending— Federal and National

JOSEPH R. ANTOS AND ALICE M. RIVLIN

The fact that Americans are spending a growing portion of their income for health care and will spend even more in the future is not necessarily alarming. However, it forces us to face two important questions: How can we be sure we are getting our money's worth? And how will we pay the health care bill? Before we tackle those questions we must understand health care spending trends as well as possible. In this chapter we focus on the growth of the federal government's spending for health care and why we believe it to be unsustainable. We also show that the federal dilemma is just a piece of the bigger picture: total spending on health care is growing rapidly, both in the United States and elsewhere in the world. The two challenges are closely intertwined.

Federal health spending, estimated to be about $676 billion in 2006,[1] is dominated by two major entitlement programs primarily benefiting senior citizens. The largest, Medicare, pays for hospital and physician care and prescription drugs for seniors and the disabled. The other, Medicaid, is a joint federal-state program that provides health coverage for low-income people. About two-thirds of Medicaid spending is devoted to

Figure 1-1. *Composition of Federal Spending, 2006 Projection*

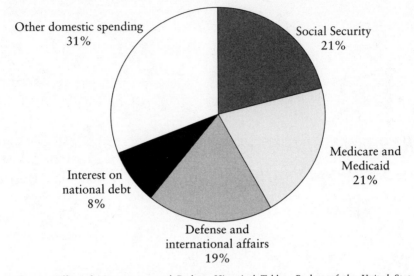

Other domestic spending
31%

Social Security
21%

Medicare and
Medicaid
21%

Interest on
national debt
8%

Defense and
international affairs
19%

Source: Office of Management and Budget, Historical Tables, *Budget of the United States Government: Fiscal Year 2006* (Government Printing Office, 2006).

health care for the elderly and disabled.[2] Federal spending on these two programs alone is estimated at $538 billion in 2006—more than defense and about the same as Social Security (figure 1-1).[3] This amount is 21 percent of the federal budget, and nearly 35 percent of everything Americans spend for health care.[4]

If current trends continue, Medicare and Medicaid will grow considerably faster than Social Security and far more rapidly than federal revenues at current tax rates. The Congressional Budget Office (CBO) projects that by 2050 the continuation of current trends in medical spending per capita combined with the aging of the population could drive spending for these two entitlements alone to 22 percent of total national spending.[5] That is more than the proportion of total national spending currently allocated to *all* federal programs. In other words, to pay for Medicare and Medicaid in 2050, the rest of the government would have to close down completely or the size of government and the taxes that pay for it would have to increase greatly. Without a radical change in attitudes toward taxes and the role of government, current trends are clearly unsustainable.

Such mechanical trend projections are mindless. By definition, unsustainable growth is bound to slow. Nevertheless, they illustrate some important points. First, future growth in overall federal spending depends almost entirely on decisions about federal health benefits. Other spending programs, including Social Security, will have far less impact on future budgets. Second, the growth of federal spending for Medicare and Medicaid will force stark budgetary choices in the future, even if their rates of growth slow considerably. Tax revenues under the current tax system rise as the economy grows, but not much faster. If spending for federal health care continues to rise substantially faster than tax revenues do, policymakers will have to cut deeply and continuously into all other federal spending or raise tax rates continuously, or both. These stark choices dramatize the importance of exploring ways to slow the growth of federal health spending.

Not Just a Federal Budget Problem

The federal budget dilemma dramatically illustrates the far more fundamental fact that Americans devote a high proportion of their total spending to health care and that the proportion is growing. That spending now totals more than 16 percent of gross domestic product (GDP), up from only 7 percent in 1970. The President's Council of Economic Advisors projects that under current trends health spending will exceed 20 percent of all American spending by 2015 (figure 1-2). In other words, if health care spending rises at historical rates, it will grow as a share of everyone's budgets—public and private. That is not necessarily a bad thing. The medical professions are more and more effective in curing disease and extending life, and Americans may well feel that health care is an increasingly desirable expenditure. But the rising share of income devoted to health will force families and businesses, as well as governments, to make difficult choices between health care and other priorities, such as education, housing, and environmental protection.

Moreover, if they are going to spend an ever-increasing portion of their total income on health care, Americans will want to be sure they are getting their money's worth. The American health care delivery system has many strong points. Wealthy foreigners, who could afford to go

Figure 1-2. *National Health Expenditures as a Percentage of GDP*

Percentage of GDP

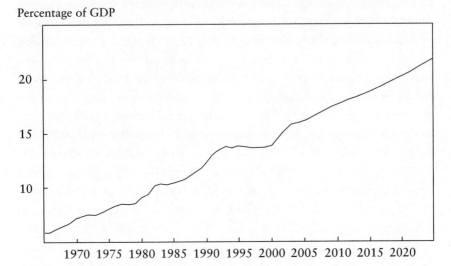

Source: U.S. Department of Health and Human Services, Centers for Medicare & Medicaid Services, Office of the Actuary, "National Health Care Expenditures Projections: 2005–2015"; Council of Economic Advisers.

anywhere in the world for treatment, often seek care in the best American hospitals to get the benefit of the world's most advanced treatment techniques and technology. But the American system has serious downsides as well. It delivers care of uneven quality at high average cost compared with other countries and leaves some 46 million people without health care insurance.[6]

Such shortcomings complicate the problem of reducing the growth of federal health programs. If the federal health budget were the only concern, the problem would be conceptually simple: the growth of federal health care spending could be slowed by reducing benefits, reimbursement rates, or eligibility for federal programs. For example, the types of health benefits paid for by Medicaid could be narrowed or the minimum age for Medicare could be raised. But such actions would only shift costs to the private sector and other levels of government, likely increase the number of people without health care coverage, and do nothing to improve the quality of care or the efficiency of delivery. Hence, the challenge to federal decisionmakers is to find ways of moderating the rise of federal health spending that move the whole system toward higher quality, greater efficiency, broader coverage, and slower overall health spending growth.

Most providers of health care are affected by both federal and non-federal health spending and policies. Patients move back and forth between public and private health insurance as their age and circumstances change, and many people have both types of insurance. Hence federal programs play a pivotal role in the health system and often exert considerable influence on the rest of the system. For example, Medicare's shift to prospective payments for hospitals in the 1980s appears to have accelerated the shortening of hospital stays, not just for Medicare patients but for other patients. Since federal health care spending is large and growing, the federal government has the potential to exert leadership and leverage on the rest of the health care delivery system. In this book we try to answer the question: can federal health care programs be reformed in ways that slow their future spending growth and move the whole health care system toward greater efficiency, effectiveness, and fairness?

Why Health Care Spending Is Growing So Fast— Here and Elsewhere

Americans devote a larger proportion of their total spending to health care than do other advanced countries, but they do not have better health outcomes to show for this higher spending. In 2003, when the United States was devoting 15 percent of its GDP to health, the average for Organization for Economic Cooperation and Development (OECD) countries—30 democracies located mainly in Europe and North America—was 8.8 percent. In Switzerland, the next highest spender after the United States, health expenditures represented 11.5 percent of GDP, while several other wealthy countries of western Europe, together with Canada, spent around 10 percent of their GDP for health, and Japan and the United Kingdom spent less than 8 percent (table 1-1).[7] These countries have populations that are aging faster than the U.S. population, and their health outcomes—measured by life expectancy, infant mortality, and other measures—are considerably better than those of Americans.

The reasons for the higher level of spending on health care in the United States are varied and not totally understood. Despite its higher

Table 1-1. *OECD Health Spending and Outcomes, 2003*

Country	Health spending as percentage of GDP	Life expectancy (years)	Infant mortality (deaths per 1,000 live births)
United States	15.0	77.2	6.9
Switzerland	11.5	80.4	4.3
Canada	9.9	79.7	5.4
Japan	7.9	81.8	3.0
United Kingdom	7.7	78.5	5.3
OECD average	8.8	77.8	6.1

Source: Organization for Economic Cooperation and Development, *Health at a Glance: OECD Indicators 2005* (Paris, 2005).

spending, the United States lags behind many other advanced countries on measures of utilization of health resources. In 2003 the United States had fewer practicing physicians, fewer nurses, and fewer days spent in acute care hospital beds per capita than the median advanced country.[8] Expensive equipment, such as CT scanners and MRI devices, which used to be more widely available in the United States than in other advanced countries, now seem to be at least equally prevalent in European countries.[9] Part of the difference is attributable to more intensive treatment of some conditions, for example, more joint replacements for arthritis and more by-pass surgeries to improve heart functioning. Part is because of higher costs of treatment in the U.S. health system. The United States pays higher compensation to doctors and other highly skilled medical personnel, higher prices for hospital stays, and higher drug costs than most other developed countries.[10] The highly complex and fragmented American health care delivery system also generates very high administrative costs. In 2003 total health administrative costs in the United States were estimated to be $111 billion; these costs are growing at a rate of 11.2 percent annually and are projected to double, to $223 billion, by 2012.[11] Higher health care expenses do allow Americans greater choice of health providers, quicker access to the newest drugs and treatments, and a variety of care management approaches—but the cost may be higher than necessary.

Despite their lower level of health spending, other advanced countries are also experiencing rapid growth in their health care spending. From 1992 to 1997, growth in health expenditures in OECD member countries

Figure 1-3. *Growth in GDP and Health Expenditures, 1992–2003*

Real annual growth (percent)

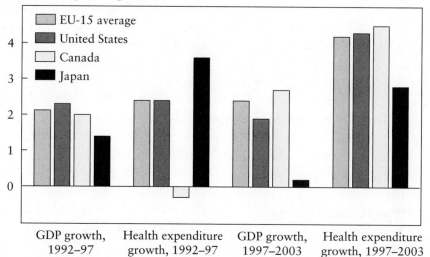

Source: OECD, *Health at a Glance: OECD Indicators 2005.*

closely matched economic growth, in part the result of deliberate efforts in the United States and Europe to contain health costs. In the late 1990s, however, health expenditures surged, substantially outpacing GDP growth. The fifteen original members of the European Union (EU-15) experienced on average a 4.2 percent increase in health expenditures from 1997 to 2003, compared with average GDP growth of 2.4 percent.[12] During this same time period, U.S. health expenditures grew 4.3 percent, more than double the 1.9 percent growth in GDP. Health expenditures also grew more rapidly than GDP in Canada (4.5 percent compared with 2.7 percent) and Japan (2.8 percent compared with 0.2 percent) (figure 1-3).[13]

Common forces are pushing health spending to higher levels in all industrial countries. First, rapid medical innovation has made medical care far more effective. More efficacious drugs and innovative medical and surgical techniques are prolonging life and curing diseases once thought to be hopeless. Many of these innovations, such as cancer treatments and joint or organ replacement, involve costly new drugs, skills, and equipment that add substantially to health care spending. Others, such as new techniques for removing cataracts, have dramatically reduced the cost of treating certain conditions. In these cases, however, the availability of cheaper and more effective interventions encourages far greater use of care. Total spending for the procedure often rises even when the cost per patient is plummeting. Second, rising incomes have increased the demand for care. With more discretionary income, people increase their health care spending. Moreover, while health care prices have been rising rapidly, third-party payment (by the government or insurer) of most of the bill reduces the impact of price on demand. Third, demographic shifts increase the demand for care. People are living longer in all advanced countries, and older people tend to use more care. For all of these reasons, the rapid rise in health care spending is a problem facing all advanced countries, even those that currently have lower average health care spending than the United States.

Increasing the efficiency of the American health care delivery system might not change the underlying forces pushing health care spending upward over the longer term. Getting waste out of the system, however, would mitigate near-term rates of growth, reduce the extent to which other priorities have to be sacrificed for health care, and reassure taxpayers and private payers that they are getting value for dollars expended.

Federal Spending for Health Care

Medicare and Medicaid dominate federal spending for health care (figure 1-4). Spending under both programs has been growing rapidly in recent decades and is projected to grow faster as the baby boom generation reaches retirement age, the proportion of older beneficiaries continues to increase, and per beneficiary spending continues to rise. The recent expansion of Medicare to include a prescription drug benefit has added to the budgetary demands made by that program.

Medicare and Medicaid are both entitlement programs. In other words, spending in a given year is determined by the number of people entitled to benefits, the health services covered under the program, and the cost of those services. Entitlement spending (sometimes called mandatory spending) is automatically funded in the budget unless Congress takes action to change the law governing who is eligible, what is covered,

Figure 1-4. *Federal Outlays for Health Programs in 2006*

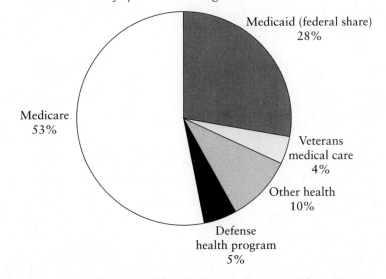

Source: OMB, Historical Tables, *Budget of the United States Government: Fiscal Year 2006.*

or how providers are reimbursed. Reducing benefits, eligibility, or reimbursement invites enormous political opposition and is infrequently
attempted. Hence, quasi-automatic entitlement spending tends to drive
out spending for programs—defense, national parks, education, and the
like—that are funded with annual appropriations. Since Medicare and
Medicaid benefit seniors, and seniors are a strong political force, the entitlement nature of these programs tends to increase the share of federal
spending devoted to older people.[14] In 1970 the joint share of Medicare
and Medicaid in the federal budget was 5.2 percent; in 2000 this share
had jumped to 18.4 percent of federal outlays. By the end of this decade,
these two programs alone are projected to make up over 25 percent of
total federal outlays (table 1-2).

Moreover, the same phenomenon plays out in state capitols. Medicaid,
which is a joint federal-state program, is the fastest-growing item in state
budgets and threatens to displace other state spending. The federal
matching formula, which makes each additional state Medicaid dollar
cost the state 50 cents or less, adds to the incentives for spending growth.
In 2004 Medicaid represented on average 16.9 percent of states' general

Table 1-2. *Increasing Health Entitlement Program*
Share of Federal Outlays, 1970–2010

Percentage of federal outlays

Program	1970	1980	1990	2000	2010
Medicaid	1.6	2.3	3.2	6.5	10.5
Medicare	3.6	5.6	8.7	11.9	15.7
Total	5.2	7.9	11.9	18.4	26.2

Source: Congressional Budget Office, "A 125-Year Picture of the Federal Government's Share of the Economy, 1950 to 2075," Long-Range Fiscal Policy Brief no. 1 (CBO: June 14, 2002, revised July 3, 2002).

fund expenditures, making it the second highest such expenditure behind elementary and secondary education (figure 1-5).

In addition to Medicare and Medicaid, other federal health programs face spending pressures. These programs include the health programs of the Department of Defense and the Veterans Administration (VA), research programs of the National Institutes of Health (NIH), and public health programs, such as the Centers for Disease Control and Prevention (see figure 1-4). Increasing demand for VA health care by veterans has led to cost overruns, and the rising cost of health care for the military is also a concern. After doubling NIH funding levels in the past few years, the recent proposal for level funding has been criticized as unduly restricting federal health research. Funding for studies of the effectiveness of health care services has been modest (compared with the cost of health care), despite the growing realization that public and private health insurance pays for both effective and ineffective treatments.

Moreover, not all federal subsidies for health care involve federal spending. Subsidies administered through the tax system place considerable pressure on the revenue side of the budget. The exclusion from income and payroll taxes of employer contributions for health insurance premiums represented more than $225 billion in forgone tax revenues in 2006.[15] These tax preferences are in effect entitlements, automatically increasing as health costs rise without explicit discussion or decisions by policymakers.

Projections of Federal Health Care Spending

Projections of past trends show spending for the three biggest federal entitlements—Social Security, Medicare, and Medicaid—rising rapidly in the

Figure 1-5. *General Fund Expenditures, 2004*

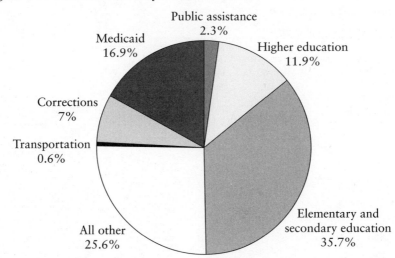

Source: National Association of State Budget Officers, "State Expenditure Report 2004" (Washington, 2005).

future.[16] Since these programs reflect promises to the elderly, the primary reason for their projected growth is often assumed to be demographic: that is, the retirement of the large baby boom population and lengthening life expectancy. However, demographics actually account for a fairly small part of the anticipated increases. The growth of Social Security spending—which is dominated by demographic changes—is projected to be relatively modest and temporary compared with projected growth of health care entitlements. If all benefits promised to current and future beneficiaries under Social Security were paid, spending under the program would rise from about 4 percent of GDP to about 6 percent and then level off as the baby-boom generation passes from the scene. Medicaid and Medicare, by contrast, are projected to continue to grow faster than Social Security and faster than federal revenues. How much faster depends on assumptions about the extent to which the growth in health spending nationally exceeds the growth in total spending.

Over the last four decades health spending has grown about 2.5 percentage points faster than the economy.[17] If these excess growth rates continue, Medicare and Medicaid alone would exceed the historic average of

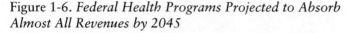

Figure 1-6. *Federal Health Programs Projected to Absorb Almost All Revenues by 2045*

Percentage of GDP

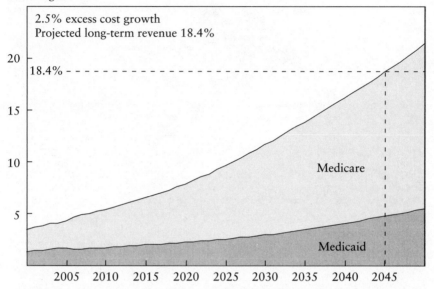

Source: Congressional Budget Office, "The Long-Term Budget Outlook" (December 2005), Appendix: Scenario 1.

total federal revenues sometime in the 2040s (figure 1-6). Although health spending slowed relative to GDP during the mid-1990s, the growth of National Health Expenditures (NHE) accelerated compared with GDP growth at the start of the twenty-first century, with an average differential of 3.3 percentage points between 2000 and 2004.[18]

As long as health spending is growing faster than other spending, the share of GDP devoted to health will rise. However, if the rate of excess health spending were less than the historical average—say 2 percentage points faster or 1.5 percentage points faster than GDP growth—pressure on the federal budget would be less. Slowing down health spending growth would make it far easier to finance the promises made to seniors under Medicare and Medicaid. One objective of this volume is to explore policies that could make such a slowdown a reality.

Other purchasers of health care services will also face rising costs if current trends continue, and that will have further consequences for the

Figure 1-7. *CBO Historical and Projected Components*

Percentage of GDP

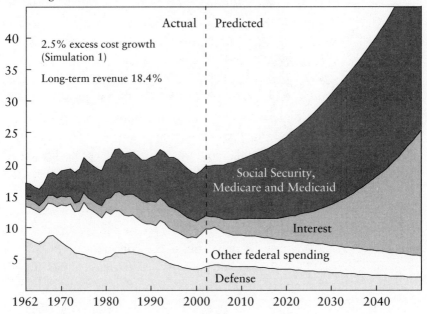

Source: CBO, "The Long-Term Budget Outlook."

budget. Employers will see escalating health costs for active employees and retirees, which translates into ever-larger tax expenditures. States also will face serious budget crunches attributable to Medicaid and state-only health programs (including public health programs).

Why Federal Health Care Spending Increases are Unsustainable

The increase in federal health care spending is not new. Indeed, since the mid-1960s, when Medicare and Medicaid were enacted, health spending has been growing faster than other spending. As may be seen in figure 1-7, the three major entitlements have risen rapidly as a share of GDP, while the share of other spending has declined. The fact that defense spending fell as the cold war wound down facilitated increases in the major entitlement programs without increases in total spending as a share of GDP.

But projected increases in health spending cannot be accommodated by cutting other spending—there simply is not enough other spending left. Nor can increases in health spending of the projected magnitudes be financed by continuous borrowing or continuous tax increases. Large sustained deficits will require devoting larger and larger portions of federal revenue just to servicing federal debt. Upward pressure on interest rates will retard economic growth. Policies intended to reduce those deficits may have their own adverse economic side effects. Big tax increases might increase revenues initially, but they can also discourage work and investment, which could have negative long-term consequences. Poorly designed program reductions might only shift the burden of health spending away from the federal government to other payers, rather than increasing the efficiency of the health system.

Policymakers cannot simply tax their way out of the problem. While taxes may well rise to subsidize the health care of a growing cohort of older and low-income people, they cannot rise continuously to cover a permanent excess of health spending growth over revenues. Similarly, policymakers cannot simply shift the excess cost burden to states or to private payers, who will also face rising health costs and limited resources. As a society we must seek ways to slow the growth of federal health care spending while promoting better value for that expenditure. A plausible approach is to use the leverage of federal spending and influence to transform the whole health care system in ways that lead to more cost-effective spending, better care, and a slower rate of spending growth.

Turning Crisis into Opportunity

Rising federal spending for health care creates a looming budget crisis that cannot be resolved with conventional tools. However, it also creates an opportunity to reform the whole national health system in ways that make it more efficient and effective. The realization that federal health spending is indeed exploding and cannot easily be cut without exacerbating pressure on the nonfederal sector may change the political dynamic and the system's tolerance for change. In the next chapter we explore options for reforming federal programs in ways that will put the whole health care system onto a more sustainable track.

Notes

1. Office of Management and Budget, *Budget of the United States Government: Fiscal Year 2006* (Government Printing Office, 2006), Historical Tables.

2. Kaiser Commission on Medicaid and Uninsured estimates, in Diane Rowland, "Medicaid at Forty," *Health Care Financing Review* 27 (Winter 2005-2006): 63–77.

3. Office of Management and Budget, Historical Tables.

4. Office of Management and Budget, Historical Tables; U.S. Department of Health and Human Services, Centers for Medicare & Medicaid Services, Office of the Actuary, "National Health Expenditures Projections: 2005–2015" (www.cms.hhs.gov/NationalHealthExpendData/downloads/proj2005.pdf).

5. Congressional Budget Office, "The Long-Term Budget Outlook" (December 2005), Appendix: Scenario 1: Higher Spending/Lower Revenues.

6. U.S. Census Bureau, "Income, Poverty, and Health Insurance Coverage in the United States, 2005," *Current Population Reports* (GPO, August 2006): 20–21.

7. Organization for Economic Cooperation and Development, *Health at a Glance: OECD Indicators 2005* (Paris, 2005).

8. Gerard F. Anderson, Bianca K. Frogner, Roger A. Johns, and Uwe E. Reinhardt, "Health Care Spending and Use of Information Technology in OECD Countries," *Health Affairs* 25 (May-June 2006): 819–31.

9. Gerard F. Anderson, Peter S. Hussey, Bianca K. Frogner, and Hugh R. Waters, "Health Spending in the United States and the Rest of the Industrialized World," *Health Affairs* 24 (July-August 2005): 903–14.

10. Uwe E. Reinhardt, Peter S. Hussey, and Gerard F. Anderson, "U.S. Health Care Spending in an International Context," *Health Affairs* 23 (May-June 2004): 10–25; Anderson and others, "Health Care Spending and Use of Information Technology."

11. Karen Davis, and Barbara S. Cooper of the Commonwealth Fund, "American Health Care: Why So Costly?" Testimony before the Senate Appropriations Subcommittee, June 11, 2003.

12. These fifteen countries—Austria, Belgium, Denmark, Finland, France, Germany, Greece, Ireland, Italy, Luxembourg, Netherlands, Portugal, Spain, Sweden, and the United Kingdom—are, on average, wealthier and have more developed economies than the ten countries that joined the EU in 2004.

13. OECD, *Health at a Glance: OECD Indicators 2005.*

14. Medicaid is a means-tested program that benefits low-income children (and some parents), the elderly, and disabled adults. Although children make up 48 percent of Medicaid enrollees and seniors only 9 percent, according to government data for 2004, seniors take up 26 percent of Medicaid expenditures, while children take up only 19 percent of expenditures. See Kaiser Commission on Medicaid and the Uninsured estimates in Diane Rowland, "Medicaid at Forty."

15. Personal communication with John Sheils. Estimation methodology based on John Sheils and Randall Haught, "The Cost of Tax-Exempt Health Benefits in 2004," *Health Affairs* web exclusive, February 25, 2004: W4-106–W4-112.

16. CBO, "The Long-Term Budget Outlook."

17. "The Long-Term Budget Outlook" prepared by the Congressional Budget Office in 2005 documents an average annual growth in national health expenditures that was 2.6 percentage points higher than growth of the economy as a whole between 1960 and 2003.

18. National Health Expenditures stayed stable as a percentage of GDP from 1993 to 2000, then began rising rapidly again. See Centers for Medicare & Medicaid Services, "National Health Care Expenditures Projections: 2005–2015."

2

Strategies for Slowing the Growth of Health Spending

JOSEPH R. ANTOS AND ALICE M. RIVLIN

Health spending in the United States is high relative to other countries and rising rapidly, but many Americans perceive they are not getting their money's worth, and tens of millions are not covered by health insurance of any kind. As chapter 1 illustrated, federal health spending, especially spending on Medicare and Medicaid, is clearly on an unsustainable track. But cutting Medicare and Medicaid benefits and restricting eligibility will shift the financial burden of health care to other payers and increase the ranks of the uninsured without improving the effectiveness of care or slowing the growth of total health spending significantly.

In this chapter we focus on how federal programs could provide leadership that will bring about positive change in the whole health system. What reforms would slow the growth of total health spending and move the whole health care system in the direction of greater efficiency and effectiveness, broader coverage, and better health outcomes? This is a tall order!

Is Comprehensive Reform Necessary to Slow Spending Growth?

Many health policy analysts believe that the United States will have little success in slowing the growth of health spending until it undertakes comprehensive reform of its complex and fragmented health system. Advocates of a strong government role in health care believe that slowing the growth of health care spending would be a far more feasible task in a simpler, more unified system covering most or all of the population. In that view, a universal system with a single payer—or even a small number of competing payers—would be in a far stronger position to cap spending, negotiate payment rates with providers, insist on efficient delivery, or refuse to pay for marginally effective services. In contrast, supporters of competitive reform argue that efficiency can be achieved by giving consumers choice and financial incentives, providing the tools for informed decisionmaking, and providing subsidies to those in need. Such an approach would reduce unnecessary spending, promote high quality care, and better meet the demands of individuals for a health system that works.

However, comprehensive reform of any sort will take either a crisis that forces widespread recognition of the need for sweeping change or national leadership willing to invest enormous political capital in working out the necessary compromises among diverse vested interests. Neither will happen quickly. In the meantime, rising health spending will likely put increasing upward pressure on federal and state budgets and cause retrenchments in public spending and employer health coverage that will leave more people uninsured.

The authors of this volume believe comprehensive reform is necessary—although they may differ on what form it should take. They also believe that the nation cannot wait for comprehensive health reform to address the problem of rising spending in as many ways as possible. Squeezing waste and inefficiency out of the system and putting in place mechanisms to make health spending more effective can set the stage for more comprehensive reform. We believe that many different approaches to improving efficiency and slowing health spending growth should be tried simultaneously. In the rest of this chapter we offer a comprehensive menu of specific reforms, all of which merit attention.

We have not attempted to estimate the potential cost savings of the options described below. Many of the policy options are in early stages of development and their likely impact on health spending cannot be gauged. Many proposals would interact with others, sometimes reinforcing and sometimes reducing their impact on cost, quality, and access to care. The net impact of any policy reform depends on the specific options that are adopted and how well they are implemented. In addition, we have not prescribed a single best course of action to reform federal health programs. As we argue below, the health system is a mix of market and regulatory elements. A realistic reform strategy would include both market-oriented and regulatory policy initiatives.

No Easy Answers

The debate on health care reform sometimes sounds like a contest over which "silver bullet" will solve the whole problem—or a big part of it— by offering better health care at lower cost for everyone. For example, the impressive contributions of information technology to reducing cost and improving quality in other sectors have generated a widely held hope that information technology can greatly increase productivity in the health sector. The common sense observation that avoiding illness saves a trip to the doctor has been translated into the hope that a nation of couch potatoes can adopt healthier lifestyles, resulting in billions saved because disease has been prevented. Multimillion-dollar awards in malpractice cases that seem out of proportion to the actual harm have raised hopes that legal reforms could substantially reduce the cost of health care. Evidence that treatment of the same diagnosis varies greatly in intensity and cost among providers—without observable differences in outcomes—has generated enthusiasm for "evidence-based medicine" and "pay-for-performance" and created a hope that aligning health reimbursement to outcomes can result in higher quality at lower cost.

All of these prescriptions have merit, but none is a silver bullet. Information technology does have potential to reduce errors and save costs in health care, but the required investment is high, and much of the benefit would come from revolutionizing the way hospitals, physicians, and other providers organize their work—not a quick or easy task. Prevention is, indeed, better than cure, but people cling tenaciously to bad health habits such as smoking and overeating. Moreover, healthier folks use medical care over a longer lifetime and do not necessarily spend less in the long run. Limits on damage claims can reduce malpractice premiums significantly in certain specialties, but their effects on overall health costs are marginal. Similarly, while evidence-based medicine and pay-for-performance are promising approaches, the needed evidence and performance measures do not now exist. A major multiyear effort will be necessary to move the health system toward rewarding performance.

In short, the prospect of a simple solution to the health spending crisis is dim. Slowing the growth of health spending will require multiple policy interventions and persistent effort to address the serious problems of our health system. Everyone—patient, provider, employer, taxpayer—will ultimately be involved in the difficult decisions necessary to slow the growth of spending to a sustainable rate.

The Problem of Third-Party Payment

When spending on video games or espresso drinks soars, no one tries to design policies to second guess consumers and slow such spending. Society relies on the price mechanism to keep supply and demand in balance and ensure reasonably efficient production. But health care is often necessary to life and health. Denying care to someone who needs it but cannot pay is widely regarded as cruel and unconscionable, especially in an emergency or with respect to a life-threatening condition. Moreover, the need for health care is often unpredictable and comes in large lumps, for example, when the patient suffers a heart attack, stroke, or serious accident. People naturally want protection from sudden, involuntary bills that could bankrupt them.

These characteristics have led to third-party payment for most health services. Many countries have national health programs paid out of tax revenues. The United States has a complex system of private and public health coverage. Many workers and their families obtain health insurance through their employers, an arrangement that is subsidized through the income tax. Seniors and the disabled are covered by Medicare, and many of the poor are eligible for Medicaid or the State Children's Health

Insurance Program (SCHIP).[1] Some people purchase their own insurance without employer help, but about 16 percent of Americans go without health insurance, either paying for care directly, receiving charity care, or going without care.

When a third party—whether the government or a private insurer—is paying for care, the patient has little incentive to consider the price or find the most efficient provider. Providers who know that the patient is not paying the bill also have little inducement to economize. This phenomenon, known as moral hazard, results in higher spending for health care than would have occurred if the patient had paid the full cost directly.[2]

Moral hazard can be diminished by requiring that patients pay more of the cost of their care out of their own pockets or by limiting the use of health services through administrative mechanisms. Raising the deductible amount that must be paid before insurance kicks in, or increasing the co-payments or coinsurance that patients pay when they receive a health service, increases cost-awareness on the part of patients and discourages the use of health services. However, even modest co-pays and deductibles may cause hardship to low-income people. If they subsequently stop taking their medications or seeking care, chronic conditions may worsen, leading to more aggressive treatment and higher costs.

Alternatively, health plans may reduce the impact of moral hazard by directly limiting access to services. Managed care plans often require patients to get a referral from a "gate-keeper" physician before accessing specialist services. Direct limits on the use of services can be effective in controlling spending, but they are unpopular with patients and providers. During the early 1990s many employers turned to managed care plans because they offered comprehensive coverage for lower premiums. Complaints from workers coupled with a booming economy and tight labor markets caused a backlash against managed care, with employers shifting back to less-managed types of insurance coverage.

Public subsidies have encouraged the purchase of private insurance or provided public health coverage to millions of people, but they have also contributed substantially to the rapid growth of health spending. Only about 25 percent of seniors had comprehensive hospital insurance in 1963; virtually all seniors gained that coverage with the implementation of Medicare in 1966.[3] Similarly, many low-income persons were given expanded access to care when Medicaid was enacted. Those programs have helped to improve the health status of seniors and the poor, but they also have added a large and rapidly growing burden on federal and state budgets.

The tax system provides generous subsidies for the purchase of private health insurance. In 2006 more than 170 million people will take advantage of federal and state tax preferences for employer-sponsored insurance worth $225 billion in reduced income and payroll taxes.[4] Tax expenditures for health care are essentially entitlements, growing automatically every year without any necessary intervention by Congress. However, they receive less attention than the spending-side entitlements, Medicare and Medicaid.

Nearly the entire amount of that tax expenditure comes from the exclusion of employer premium contributions from the taxable income of workers.[5] Although the tax exclusion helps millions of people buy health insurance, it also leads to higher spending on health insurance and promotes insurance that covers more services with lower out-of-pocket cost to be paid by consumers. Employer contributions to premiums also reduce the apparent cost of insurance even though such contributions are ultimately paid by the workers, whose wages grow less rapidly than they otherwise would. Consequently, employer-sponsored insurance tends to offer more generous coverage, which blunts the consumer's sensitivity to health care prices and encourages greater use of services.

Consumers directly paying only a fraction of the cost of their care are apt to use services that are not worth as much as they cost. The cost of additional care induced by this moral hazard effect of insurance is reflected eventually in higher insurance premiums. By promoting generous coverage, tax incentives help fuel the escalation of health care costs and insurance premiums.

The tax exclusion does not help people who are not working or who work for a firm that does not offer health insurance coverage, regardless of their income or health status. Among workers who benefit, those with higher incomes stand to gain more from the exclusion than lower-income workers. After income and payroll taxes, a high earner could save as much as 50 cents for every dollar spent on health insurance premiums, at the margin. In contrast, a low earner might save as little as 3 cents on the dollar for employer-sponsored insurance.[6]

Combining program spending for Medicare and Medicaid with the health tax expenditures, federal and state governments will devote over $875 billion to health care in 2006 and substantially larger amounts in the future. Much of that money is not spent efficiently, resulting in health care that does not return full value for the investment.

Seeking Efficient and Effective Care

Despite enormous advances in scientific knowledge, medicine remains more an art than a science. Diagnosing a patient can be difficult if he or she has multiple conditions or uncommon diseases. The choice of treatment can be complicated because different patients with a particular disease may respond well or poorly to the same therapy. Physicians may well disagree about the best treatment approach for a challenging patient. Since physicians share experience and influence each other, it is not surprising that there are substantial variations among locations and providers in how particular diagnoses are treated.

Nonetheless, the variation in medical practice across the country is much larger than one might expect to arise purely from different mixes of patients or traditions of practice. Dr. Jack Wennberg and colleagues at the Center for Evaluative Clinical Sciences at the Dartmouth Medical School have long experience analyzing Medicare data to uncover variations in resources used to treat the same diagnoses among regions, states, and providers, as well as the outcomes associated with those treatments.

Three robust results emerge from this body of research and analysis. First, the variations in resource use are huge. For example, Medicare spending for the average patient living in Miami is about two and a half times larger than it is in Minneapolis, even accounting for health and demographic differences between the two populations.[7] A study of Medicare patients suffering from one or more serious chronic diseases showed that in the last six months of life such patients averaged more than sixteen days in the hospital in New York and Hawaii, but less than eight days in Utah and Oregon. In the last two years of life, Medicare spent an average of $40,000 on such patients in New Jersey and only $25,000 in Ohio.[8]

Second, resource use is sensitive to supply. In areas with more hospital beds per capita, Medicare patients were more likely to be hospitalized, and in areas with more cardiologists per capita, Medicare patients with heart disease had more cardiologist visits.

Third, and most surprising, more aggressive treatment styles and higher spending levels do not result in better patient outcomes. One study that followed three cohorts of Medicare patients (who were hospitalized for hip fracture, colorectal cancer, and heart attack) found that greater care intensity was associated with increased mortality rates.[9] However, all is not well in low-spending areas: both high- and low-cost areas underutilize effective services, such as mammography or vaccination for pneumonia.

These findings reflect a disturbing variability in efficiency in the health system. They suggest that finding ways to make practices of the least efficient providers more like the most efficient would save large amounts of resources, both in Medicare and in the rest of the health system.

The challenge is moving from documenting inefficiency to reducing it without doing more harm than good. Information on what works in health care (and for whom) is inadequate, and providers often fail to use available information on effective medicine. Fee-for-service payment encourages greater resource use and rewards excessive treatment and even medical errors. Medicare, for example, will pay for the readmission of a patient to a hospital to treat an infection acquired in that hospital.

Major efforts are under way to address the lack of information on effective treatment. New data sources are being developed, including information from insurance claim records and patient registries that can provide evidence of how well medical interventions work in day-to-day practice rather than under the more carefully controlled (and less realistic) conditions of clinical trials. Comparative effectiveness studies analyze the body of scientific literature to draw conclusions about which of several treatment strategies are the most promising. Medicare has modified its coverage process to permit payment for certain treatments (such as implantable cardiac defibrillators) on a provisional basis, contingent on the development of evidence on the success of the treatment among Medicare patients.

It is sometimes said that only 15 percent of what doctors do is backed by hard evidence.[10] That may be an exaggeration, but it is clear that the medical profession's ability to treat patients has greatly outrun its knowledge of what works best out of a growing range of options. Efforts to improve the knowledge base must become an ongoing and substantial part of the health system.

Despite the lack of clear evidence for much of what is done in medicine, the wealth of treatment options can be overwhelming even for well-trained physicians trying to keep up with medical progress. Methods being developed to help physicians manage information overload include:

—Practice guidelines based on evidence rather than subjective judgment or professional consensus;

—Disease management and other patient management methods that rely on evidence-based protocols and improved coordination among providers;

—Improved Internet access to the latest scientific studies; and

—Computer-based decision support tools.[11]

Many physicians may not make the best use of such information tools, however. Accessing computer-based information can interfere with face-to-face interaction between physician and patient. Computers are typically not available in examining rooms, for example, although hand-held devices may reduce this problem for physicians willing to use them. Although younger physicians are more comfortable with such technology, the practice style of many older physicians is incompatible with its use. In addition, most physicians typically see patients with common diseases that may be easily diagnosed, diseases that the physician has long treated in conventional ways. Conventional practice may therefore lag behind the best evidence unless new findings are brought to the physician's attention.

The business realities of running a medical practice also inhibit physician adherence to evidence-based standards. Fee-for-service payment combined with low negotiated reimbursement rates from insurers promote the use (and overuse) of health services. The patient is unlikely to object to treatment that does not meet evidence standards since he or she is largely shielded from the direct cost of care by insurance and is far less knowledgeable about treatment alternatives than the physician. The insurance system has a bias in favor of treating rather than preventing disease, even though prevention might be less expensive.

To improve the efficiency and effectiveness of health care, the knowledge base necessary for sound medical decisionmaking must be built and that knowledge made accessible and usable to patients, physicians, and payers. The financial incentives must be redirected toward more prudent use of care while also finding mechanisms that ensure that patients seek necessary care.

The Problem of the Uninsured

The American health financing system leaves about 45 million people without health insurance at any given time and larger numbers without coverage for some part of the year.[12] Perhaps as many as 60 million people are uninsured at any time during the year.[13] Over the past two decades, the number of people without health insurance has grown by 50 percent.

People without insurance have limited access to health care through public hospitals and clinics and charity care offered by private providers. As a result, the uninsured often have untreated ailments and chronic conditions. Eventually they may require aggressive and expensive medical interventions that could have been prevented with more timely and routine attention from a health provider.

The rising cost of health care is pushing more and more people into the ranks of the uninsured. As insurance premiums rise, employers pare back benefits, increase the share of costs that must be paid by employees, drop coverage altogether, or decide not to offer it in the first place. Employment-based coverage is sensitive to the business cycle, declining during periods of economic slowdown and rising during expansions. Disturbingly, the share of the population with employer coverage did not grow much above historical levels even during the record boom of the 1990s. Medicaid has proven to be a safety valve, growing as a share of the total as private insurance enrollment fell off.

The rising numbers of uninsured also add to the total cost of health care. Uninsured individuals impose a cost on everyone else when they need health care and are unable to pay. Uncompensated care could amount to as much as $35 billion annually.[14] Moreover, people without insurance tend to forgo preventive health care and delay treatment, which can cause them to suffer needlessly, lead to complications, and require more aggressive and expensive medical interventions. The uninsured tend to seek care in hospital emergency departments—an exceedingly expensive source of care.

Thus, the problem of the uninsured is not just a matter of fairness. Reducing health spending growth in ways that further adds to the ranks of the uninsured is not only inequitable; it tends to make the health system even less efficient.

Reform Strategies

Objectives of a broad system reform include slowing the growth of health spending by increasing the system's efficiency, ensuring that more people have access to health insurance, improving the availability of essential health services, providing consumers control over their health care, and promoting medical innovation. Some policy objectives are likely to be incompatible with others, requiring careful balancing of goals. However, it should be possible to make progress on a variety of objectives even as the nation works to slow spending in a $2 trillion system.

Two basic approaches dominate the running debate among experts and policymakers about the best reform strategy for the health system. Market strategy proponents argue that promoting competition and consumer choice would establish appropriate incentives for greater system efficiency and ultimately lower growth in health spending. Regulatory strategy advocates believe that stronger government action is needed to control costs directly and to police an unruly marketplace to avoid risks that individuals should not be forced to bear. Both sets of beliefs are deeply held, causing a philosophical impasse that limits the scope of policies that can be seriously considered in Congress. We argue that a blended strategy that uses both market and regulatory approaches is most likely to be successful.

Market Reform Strategy

Proponents of a market strategy believe that if individuals had more direct responsibility for the cost of their care, they would weigh these costs and the value they receive more carefully. Providers would be forced to compete for consumer dollars on the basis of price, quality, and customer service. This heightened competition would cause health care providers to adopt more efficient practice styles. Prices for services would be established in the market, reflecting both supply and demand conditions more accurately than government-set prices. Such pricing would provide incentives for continued medical innovation.

Giving consumers choices among competing health plans is not a new idea to the federal government. The Federal Employees Health Benefits Program (FEHBP) has offered federal employees and retirees a wide choice of health plans since its founding in 1960. While having a choice of health plans may make consumers more cost-conscious when they choose plans, it still leaves a third party (the plan) paying most of the bills.

Another approach that reduces the moral hazard problem would require consumers to pay out of pocket for most health expenditures, while protecting them only from the catastrophic losses that could accompany a major illness or accident. Such consumer-driven health plans typically offer insurance with a high deductible plus a savings account, to which the individual or his employer may contribute, designed to help the individual pay the out-of-pocket costs. Such plans encourage more prudent decisionmaking on the part of both patients and physicians by making both more aware of the cost of care and of the fact that consumers are using their own money to pay for that care. Congress introduced this idea into the discussion in 2003 when it enacted health savings accounts (HSAs), an idea that is discussed in more detail later.

Reliable information on the cost, quality, and appropriateness of care is needed if consumers are to make sound health care decisions. Such information is not readily available today, and the information that is available is fragmentary and difficult to interpret.

The price that the consumer will pay out of pocket for a service, for example, depends on who delivers the service and whether the consumer has satisfied his annual deductible. The cost of a full episode of care is a better indicator of cost for conditions requiring hospitalization or the services of more than one provider. However, since services are typically billed individually, ascertaining a price for the full bundle can be difficult.

Mortality rates, hospital readmission rates, and other commonly available quality indicators are inadequate assessments of provider quality and must be interpreted with care. Data comparing the effectiveness of alternative treatments are not readily available, and the typical consumer would need substantial medical knowledge or the advice of a physician to interpret the studies that do exist.

Insurers, providers, and government agencies are beginning to develop better consumer information. Many insurers have begun to experiment with ways to make price data available to consumers.[15] Aetna, for example, gives its subscribers access to physician-specific rates for 25 common services in its Cincinnati pilot project. CIGNA focuses its pricing information on outpatient procedures, such as MRI (magnetic resonance imaging), where the variation in cost is substantial and members are more likely to consider choosing a provider based on cost. The White House has urged providers to make price and quality data available to consumers,[16] and many states and the federal government make available quality indicators for hospitals, nursing homes, and other providers.

Nonetheless, critics are concerned that the average consumer is poorly equipped to interpret complex price and quality information and that high out-of-pocket costs will cause people, especially those with low incomes, to forgo both unnecessary and necessary care.[17] That could worsen health outcomes and increase costs.

Moreover, much health spending is concentrated among a small number of people with very high expenses: 10 percent of the population accounts for 69 percent of the nation's health spending.[18] Much of the spending for high-cost patients is above the deductible amount for a typical consumer-driven health plan and unaffected by financial incentives. Other methods of limiting inappropriate spending, such as care management for high-cost cases, may be more effective in controlling costs.[19]

The list of steps necessary to create a functioning health market is daunting. It includes insurance market reform, improved health information, better antitrust enforcement, malpractice reform, and restructured and better-targeted subsidies to individuals for private insurance.[20] Since such policies are controversial, and there are both political and technical disagreements over how to proceed, the task will not be easy.

Regulatory Strategy

Critics of market-based reform argue there is a social responsibility to make sure that everyone has access to good quality care when they need it. Third-party payment has become the norm precisely because consumers want, and deserve, to know that they will have the ability to pay for medical services when the need arises. Consumers, especially people who are ill, cannot become sufficiently informed on the technicalities of medical practice to make wise choices and thus are likely to be unduly influenced by providers.

Proponents of a regulatory strategy also argue that there is a social responsibility to ensure that good quality care is delivered as efficiently as possible. We cannot rely upon private companies to provide that care without regulation, as experience shows that insurers seek to avoid covering people with serious health conditions and drug companies charge substantially more than they need to cover their costs of production. Large companies will exploit their market power to the disadvantage of consumers. Moreover, large government programs have considerable market power that should be exercised on behalf of consumers and taxpayers. Proponents of stronger regulation assert that Medicare has been more successful than private insurers in slowing the growth of health spending, attributing that record to Medicare's ability to price services more aggressively.[21] Many policymakers agree with that assessment despite some evidence to the contrary.[22]

Admittedly, there are risks to setting lower prices for health services than would have prevailed in an unregulated market, since health providers may try to make up for the lower price by increasing the volume of services. For that reason, Medicare price cuts have typically resulted in less budgetary savings than might have been expected without the induced growth in the use of services.[23] Moreover, if prices are held to low levels over the long term, health providers and suppliers exit the market. The unwillingness of many providers to accept the low reimbursements under Medicaid reduces options for low-income people enrolled in the program, and some providers limit the number of Medicare patients they see.

Proponents of regulation argue that just because regulation has sometimes been carried out stupidly does not mean it cannot be done well.

They envision a system of universal health coverage in which the government uses its power to ensure that health services are effective and delivered efficiently. This could involve analyzing data to establish best practices, promulgating practice guidelines, and refusing to pay for care that did not conform to those guidelines, as well as imposing caps on total health spending and devising rules for enforcing those caps.

Blended Strategy

In fact, America's health system is a hodgepodge of market and regulatory elements that have accreted over decades. Replacing this complex, hybrid system with either a pure market system or pure regulated system seems both unlikely and unworkable. Realistically, moving the current health system toward greater efficiency as well as equity will take a blend of market-oriented and regulatory reforms.

An example of a blended strategy would be aggressive implementation of pay for performance by both public and private payers. Such a strategy would recognize the basic tenet of the market model that informed consumers will seek out providers who offer the best value in terms of price, quality, and customer service. But it also recognizes that, as long as a large fraction of health spending is covered by insurance, the most important decisions about what and where to buy are made by third-party payers, not individual consumers. Employers have taken steps to promote more informed purchasing by their employees. For example, the Leapfrog Group of large employers has received public acclaim for its efforts to reward doctors and hospitals for improving the quality, safety, and affordability of health care, and to help consumers reap the benefits of making smart health care decisions. Medicare also has begun experimenting with ways to provide stronger financial incentives for hospitals and physicians to provide high quality care under the rubric of P4P.

Regulation and markets are facts of life in the health system. Health reform is likely to nudge the system toward either greater regulation or more competitive markets, but a wholesale shift in one direction is implausible. Policy proposals should be evaluated for their likely impact on spending, access, and quality, as well as for their longer-term influence on the balance between government and individual control.

Using Federal Programs to Lead the Way

The size and impact of federal health programs suggest that well-designed reforms of these programs can serve as a catalyst for improvements of the whole health system. Of course, the reverse is also true: Poorly conceived federal policy can make matters worse for everyone, and it can be very difficult to reverse even the most misguided federal policy once it has been implemented.

Of all federal health programs, Medicare has the greatest leverage on the day-to-day operation of the health system. As the largest single purchaser of health care, Medicare policies directly affect virtually every provider.

Since Medicare's policies have the force of law, they have enormous influence over a vast industry. Record keeping, coding, and billing practices established by Medicare are the industry norm. Medicare has introduced innovations in payment methods, such as prospective payment systems, that have been widely adopted by private insurers. Changes in the way Medicare manages or pays for benefits, as with the prescription drug benefit, can cause health plans and providers to alter the way they manage both their Medicare and private business. Medicare's recent emphasis on price transparency and quality reporting, for example, is likely to lead to greater access to such information for all consumers. Initiatives to test new ways to manage high-cost patients, to promote the use of evidence-based treatment, and other innovations have stimulated interest among private insurers and health plans in such approaches.

Innovative approaches are also being tested by states seeking to improve the operation of their Medicaid programs, which together account for as much total health spending as Medicare. Efforts to make other federal health programs—including SCHIP, the Veterans Health Administration (VHA), and the Defense Department's TRICARE program—more efficient could pay off in terms of reduced growth in federal outlays. Lessons learned from such policies can often be applied more broadly (see chapters 4 and 5). Indeed, examples of efficient practices in VHA are already influencing other systems.

The federal tax system plays a major role in subsidizing employment-based private health insurance. Restructuring the tax preference, perhaps by capping the amount that may be excluded from taxable income and providing a refundable tax credit for health insurance, could better target those in need and minimize the adverse incentives that promote inefficiency in the health system.[24]

In addition, regulatory agencies, such as the Federal Trade Commission (FTC) and the Food and Drug Administration (FDA), establish and enforce "rules of the road" for the health sector. The FTC seeks to prevent anticompetitive business practices and to protect consumers against unfair, deceptive, or fraudulent practices. In the health sector, that has meant challenges to hospital mergers and other actions to discourage anticompetitive behavior or to improve consumer knowledge. The FDA regulates drugs and medical devices to ensure safety and effectiveness. The approval of new drugs, generic versions of brand drugs, and medical devices can have substantial impacts on the treatment of disease and the cost of health care.

Research agencies, such as the National Institutes of Health (NIH) and the Agency for Healthcare Research and Quality (AHRQ), contribute to the development of medical innovation and improvements in clinical practice and the delivery of health care. Research on health system improvements, including comparative effectiveness analysis, receives relatively little funding, however, despite the large potential payoff to such work.

Policy Options

In this section, we discuss policy proposals that show promise of mitigating the projected increase in federal health spending and leading the non-federal system toward greater efficiency at the same time (see table 2-1 for a brief summary of proposals). While substantial work would be required to implement any of them, they illustrate the many possible avenues to pursue.

Setting Prices or Payment Rates

The way in which health care products and services are priced or reimbursed can determine the type of services that are provided, the quality of the resulting care, and the cost of that care. Reimbursing providers on a fee-for-service basis is widely seen as creating incentives to produce more

Table 2-1. *Reform Options for Federal Health Programs and Health-Related Activities*

Improve price setting

Pay-for-performance	Implement and evaluate reimbursement rates based on performance (P4P) in federal programs, especially Medicare.
Bidding	Design and implement bidding approaches to purchase of drugs, devices, and packages of health services in federal programs.
Leverage market share	Negotiate lower prices for medical products and services, using federal programs' market power and legal authority.

Develop information

Health information technology (IT)	Develop standards for interoperable health IT for hospitals, physicians, and other health providers. Provide incentives and low-cost financing for adoption of systems that meet the standards. Use VA health system as laboratory to test improvements in health IT, including hardware, software, and work methods. Use incentives and requirements to meet target date for implementation of universal, portable, individual medical records.
Data development	Collect and make accessible data on cost and outcomes of health treatments by diagnosis and provider, starting with Medicare database.
Research on outcomes and effectiveness	Sponsor cost-effectiveness and comparative effectiveness studies of medical treatments and disseminate results widely.

Improve health care delivery

Guidelines	Create evidence-based practice guidelines by using Medicare's "coverage with evidence development" to assess use of treatments and patients most likely to benefit. Give providers information to compare their performance against their peers and measure their adherence to practice guidelines.
Care management and coordination	Increase incentives for Medicare beneficiaries to enroll in managed care plans and participate in disease management programs. Increase incentives for providers to cooperate with disease management programs and improve coordination of patient care.
End-of-life care	Promote greater public awareness of end-of-life health issues, including importance of advance directives and understanding of treatment options.
Lower-cost delivery settings	Increase incentives for use of lower-cost treatment settings.
Health promotion and disease prevention	Support studies on cost-effectiveness of preventive health services.

Promote consumerism and competition	
Premium support	Introduce premium support in Medicare, modeled after Federal Employees Health Benefits Program.
Premium assistance	Encourage state experimentation in Medicaid to involve beneficiaries in decisions about their care, such as the "cash and counseling" demonstration.
Health savings accounts	Encourage high-deductible insurance plans tied to tax-favored health savings accounts.
Limit health outlays	
Transform Medicare and Medicaid	Convert Medicaid to indexed block grant that rewards better health outcomes and lower-cost treatment.
	Convert Medicaid and Medicare to modified entitlements, requiring Congress to vote on total spending at least every few years.
Limit tax exclusion	Cap and gradually reduce tax exclusion for employer contributions to health insurance premiums.
Other options	
Drug approvals	Streamline FDA approval process for new drugs and medical devices; develop standards for new types of generics, including follow-on biologics.
Malpractice reform	Reform tort system to reduce defensive medicine costs, improve patient safety, and promote appropriate redress for injury.

tests, procedures, and office visits, even if these services are likely to provide only minimal improvements in the patient's health. Managed care plans can be more efficient, because they have an incentive to provide only the services needed to keep the patient healthy. Medicare has not required its beneficiaries to move into managed care (although they have the option of enrolling in Medicare Advantage). Medicare has been an innovator in developing more effective pricing methods within its traditional fee-for-service system, in which the vast majority of beneficiaries are enrolled.

Medicare's first major pricing reform was the shift in 1983 from cost-based reimbursement to a prospective payment system (PPS) for hospital services. Paying a fixed amount for a given diagnosis gives hospitals an incentive to reduce unnecessary costs.[25] Consequently, lengths of stay were reduced and hospital care became more efficient, although this approach also encouraged hospitals to discharge patients to skilled nursing facilities and other providers of postacute care that is billed to Medicare. Since then, Medicare has adopted prospective payment, or a predetermined schedule of fees, for most covered services. The program has analyzed ways to refine PPS, including payment adjustments for more acutely ill patients and a single payment for a larger bundle of services (such as the inpatient stay and some period of postacute care).

Pay-for-performance (P4P) is a promising tool for promoting high-quality care and reducing unnecessary costs, although implementing such a system poses major challenges.[26] To be effective, quality measures must identify real differences in provider performance, adjusting for the severity of illness of their patients and multiple dimensions of quality care. Mortality or hospital readmission rates and patient satisfaction measure only part of the broader quality concept that a well-designed P4P program would reward. Physician acceptance of both P4P principles and the specific quality measures is essential to making this approach successful on a sustainable basis. It is not known how much money must be at stake to promote improvements in provider performance. There are questions about the capacity of poor performing physicians and hospitals to improve the quality of their care when insurers reduce their reimbursements. Medicare has the clout to advance P4P, but it must move forward carefully to avoid institutionalizing an inadequate payment formula.

P4P has proven controversial among some conservatives.[27] They argue that Medicare has so much leverage over the market that the adverse consequences of any error in assessing provider performance would be magnified greatly. The fear is that Medicare's size and regulatory authority would create a de facto federal standard of care for private insurance that would be difficult to modify, even though the science of medicine continued to evolve. One solution, according to that argument, is to prevent the use of P4P in traditional Medicare while permitting smaller private plans in Medicare Advantage to experiment with such payment systems.

While allowing traditional Medicare to develop P4P carries risks, the program should not simply ignore the adverse incentives of its current payment methods that discourage quality and efficiency. Those incentives influence medical practice regardless of who is paying the bill, and they must be addressed if systemwide improvements are to be made in care delivery.

Although a well-designed P4P system would provide financial incentives for high-quality care, even that advance would not ensure that the price level was appropriate. P4P, PPS, and other common formula-based payment systems used in Medicare may not accurately reflect the market conditions facing individual providers in local markets. At best, Medicare's payments approximate the average demand and supply conditions in each market. But that means some services and providers are overpaid, and others are underpaid. Consequently, exceptional growth in program outlays for some services appears to be motivated by distorted payment incentives.

Medicare has explored bidding approaches as an alternative to formula-based payment methods. By requiring all sellers to submit their best offer in advance, bidding approaches elicit prices that better reflect local market conditions.

Bidding has been tested for pricing durable medical equipment (such as wheelchairs, hospital beds, and oxygen equipment). Demonstration projects conducted between 1999 and 2002 in two locations found that bidding reduced program costs by about 20 percent.[28] A nationwide competitive bidding system for durable medical equipment is expected to begin in January 2007, although there are concerns that such a system will drive smaller suppliers out of business, ultimately driving prices up and reducing service to beneficiaries.

Greater controversy surrounds the decision to use bidding to set payments under the new Medicare drug benefit. Under this system, each prescription drug plan (PDP) submits a bid detailing the list of covered drugs (formulary), cost-sharing requirements (deductible, copayments, and coverage gaps), distribution network (retail and mail-order pharmacies), and the premium they propose to charge. Medicare pays an amount equal to 75 percent of the average premium, and beneficiaries pay the rest. This approach relies on the PDPs to negotiate their best price from drug manufacturers. Plans with lower costs can charge lower premiums and attract more enrollment; larger plans are in a better bargaining position to extract the greatest price concessions from manufacturers.

Critics argue that this approach fails to take advantage of Medicare's aggregate buying power. If the program negotiated on behalf of all of its beneficiaries, the resulting prices might be substantially lower than those obtained by the PDPs. The cost of producing an additional pill is generally low, which leaves room for downward price flexibility. However, drug manufacturers point out that the cost of research and testing a new drug is high and only a few drugs are financial successes. If aggressive government negotiation to lower prices to Medicare makes drug companies significantly less profitable, it could retard the creation of new pharmaceuticals.

Outside of Medicare, the government uses its market power and legal authority to extract lower drug prices than generally seen in the market. Congress requires drug manufacturers to provide rebates to state Medicaid programs, resulting in a Medicaid "best price" that is about 63 percent of the list price.[29] The Department of Veterans Affairs (VA) does even better, negotiating prices with drug manufacturers under the Federal Supply Schedule that average 53 percent of the list price, although some of the price difference is the result of not having to use retail pharmacies for distribution. Federal Supply Schedule prices are available to all direct federal purchasers of pharmaceuticals, including VA, the Defense Department, and the Public Health Service. Congress gave VA considerable leverage in its negotiations, and drug manufacturers must participate in the Federal Supply Schedule to sell their pharmaceuticals under Medicaid.

The challenge for policymakers is finding a balance between the short-term savings and the longer-term consequences of direct negotiations or other methods of setting prices administratively.

Developing Information

Any attempt to improve the efficiency of health services will require better information to be successful. Federal action can improve the knowledge base for clinical decisionmaking by promoting health information technology, developing comprehensive data on patient care, and sponsoring research on outcomes and effectiveness of care.

HEALTH INFORMATION TECHNOLOGY. More can be done to build on the health information technology (IT) activities already under way at various federal agencies. Much attention has been given to the electronic medical record (EMR) system used by VHA, which is one of the pioneers in this area. Although that system can be improved to facilitate true interoperability across sites of care, it provides a solid demonstration of the value of health IT.

The Veterans Health Information System and Technology Architecture (VistA) provides comprehensive diagnostic and treatment information for each patient as well as financial and management information. The system allows providers not only to order various services (including medications, x-rays, nursing orders, diets, and laboratory tests) but also to review detailed information on the patient and his treatment. Although providers in one facility cannot currently access EMR information on care provided in another facility, VHA is working on a system upgrade that will establish a single systemwide record that is accessible to all VA providers (see chapter 5). The successful quality improvement initiatives undertaken by VHA to date have relied in large part on the patient data available through VistA.

The Department of Health and Human Services (HHS) is heavily promoting the use of EMRs that can be linked together to enable data sharing among doctors, hospitals, and other providers, as well as patients.[30] For example, the department is developing electronic standards in conjunction with the private sector to promote the exchange of data across computer systems. The Agency for Healthcare Research and Quality is funding projects to develop interoperable health information systems at the state and regional level. The CMS (Centers for Medicare & Medicaid Services) has several demonstration projects to test how health IT can improve the quality of care, and it is modifying the VA's EMR software for the physician office setting.

A recent executive order issued by the White House directs federal health care programs—Medicare, VHA, TRICARE, the Federal Employees Health Benefit Program, and the Indian Health Service—to transition to health IT that meets interoperability standards.[31] In addition, the order requires a similar upgrading of health IT capability used by providers, health plans, and insurers who contract with those programs. Such requirements establish a more certain market for improved health IT systems and software that could spur more rapid development.

Recognizing that the cost of investing in health IT can be an insurmountable barrier for some providers, particularly small physician practices, Congress created a "safe harbor" that allows physicians to accept donations of software for EMRs or for electronic prescribing, or for information technology and training services.[32] Such donations are likely to be made by hospitals, health plans, or insurers, who might offer help with health IT to providers in whom they have a financial interest. Previously, physicians could not accept such donations because of the potential for a conflict of interest.

Patients' concerns about maintaining the privacy of their personal information, heightened after recent reports of unauthorized disclosures of patient data and other confidential information, are another barrier to the widespread use of health IT.[33] Greater technical safeguards and more enforcement are necessary.

DATA DEVELOPMENT. Sound medical decisionmaking requires a knowledge base of clinical research to ascertain what treatments are likely to be successful and under what conditions. In addition, patients need information about quality of care to make informed choices about which providers to see. Both objectives can be furthered by efforts to assemble data on the care of patients covered by federal programs.

Health IT, particularly EMRs, can provide a mechanism to efficiently collect information on patients and the course of their treatments. Ideally, a fully wired health system could monitor and analyze patient progress on a large scale, enabling more reliable judgments about the effectiveness of specific treatments and the value-added of providers. Until then, currently existing Medicare and Medicaid data offer a potentially rich source of patient information on which to base assessments of clinical effectiveness and quality of care.

The obstacles to developing a usable database from those programs are numerous. Medicare operates through regional carriers and intermediaries with access to billing records but not detailed patient records. Medicaid is operated through state agencies that do not currently share detailed information on billing and patient care with HHS. Assembling a longitudinal file that represents all of the health care a beneficiary receives through Medicare is a difficult undertaking, and combining data from Medicare and Medicaid is currently impossible. Desirable information is often in paper records and not retrievable in any practical manner for a large sample of patients.

Despite these difficulties, it is feasible to begin constructing a comprehensive patient-level database using Medicare data without waiting for full adoption of health IT. Such a data source would be a powerful analytic tool, revealing the effectiveness of medical treatments for the entire elderly patient population rather than a small sample of patients (as in most research studies). In addition, such data would reflect the practical problems of providing health care (such as physician or patient failure to follow a strict treatment protocol, or treatment delivered to patients with multiple problems). Clinical trials are more tightly controlled (typically involving patients with one disease and tight adherence to protocols) and yield evidence of the effectiveness of care under best practices, but those results may not be found in actual care settings.

Less ambitious data development would also yield valuable information. The CMS has undertaken a variety of projects to measure the quality of care offered by providers, ranging from hospital mortality data first reported in the late 1980s to the recent release of information on the amount of Medicare payments and the volume of services for thirty common elective hospital procedures.[34]

The federal government could also expand its data collection beyond Medicare and Medicaid. Federal insurance programs cover other large populations, including federal employees and retirees, veterans, and military personnel. Although there are legal, technical, and financial challenges, the government could explore partnerships with private insurers and health plans for the purpose of developing comprehensive health databases for a broad swath of individuals below the age of sixty-five.

Although it has several advantages in assembling health data, the government should provide other researchers, health plans, and insurers access to the resulting information so they can analyze the data and make judgments about effectiveness and quality.

RESEARCH OUTCOMES AND EFFECTIVENESS. The federal government spends little money on research to improve the quality, cost, efficiency, and effectiveness of our health care system. The lead federal agency for such research is the Agency for Healthcare Research and Quality, with an annual budget just over $300 million. Other agencies support health services research to some extent, but total federal outlays devoted to improving the delivery of health care are miniscule compared with the total amount spent for services.

Additional research could produce more evidence on the effectiveness of health services and knowledge of therapeutic approaches with the greatest chance of success given the patient's condition. Comparative effectiveness research can be difficult and expensive, particularly if the research uses clinical trials to test multiple treatment options. A far less costly approach synthesizes existing knowledge on a particular topic, identifying what can be concluded based on past studies while identifying gaps in knowledge.

Up-to-date analysis of a treatment's effectiveness, or the comparative effectiveness of a class of treatments, is an important input into a physician's decision to pursue a course of treatment. It is more difficult to assess whether a treatment is cost-effective.[35] That is, how good are the results likely to be and do they seem to justify the cost?

Cost-effectiveness could become an important consideration for insurers determining what services to cover. However, private insurers and public programs have been slow to adopt this approach, partly because of the paucity of reliable data on treatment effectiveness. An even greater challenge is cultural: the public and the medical profession do not seem eager to accept that resource constraints could be a reason to limit coverage for services. Whether an increase in life expectancy or quality of life is worth the cost of treatment, and who should pay for that treatment, are questions that must be viewed through the prism of personal and societal values.

The Oregon Health Plan systematically applied cost-effectiveness standards to Medicaid coverage.[36] Although that plan incorporated community views into the final list of covered treatments, the idea of making coverage decisions based on explicit resource constraints created a storm of protest about rationing health care.

More commonly, public and private insurers explicitly limit coverage to categories of medical services (such as dental services) as a contractual matter. Decisions about whether to pay for specific treatment within a covered category are typically based on the circumstances of the individual case, reflecting a medical necessity standard that may be based on common practice in the community rather than on formal analysis of scientific evidence on effectiveness. Payment denials may be appealed in many cases, and insurers may decide to pay for a service they had previously denied.

Medicare recently adopted an approach that combines speedier access to new technologies with data on treatment effectiveness or its applicability to particular patient groups. Under "coverage with evidence development," Medicare agrees to pay its share of the cost of a new treatment for patients who have a specific disease and other characteristics that make them good candidates for the treatment. Clinical evidence is collected over the course of treatment and evaluated to determine whether the coverage policy should be changed, either expanding access to the treatment or further restricting its use.[37]

Improving Health Care Delivery

Beyond creating better information on health services' effectiveness and quality of care, additional steps can be taken to improve health care delivery.

GUIDELINES. Clinical guidelines are an important tool in promoting appropriate, high quality care. They help physicians keep up with rapid advances in medical knowledge and incorporate the latest evidence into their decisions about the best course of treatment for a patient. However, even an ambitious program to develop clinical effectiveness information will leave large areas of medicine without a strong evidence basis.

The federal government can use its data development activities to generate more comprehensive clinical guidelines. Medicare and Medicaid could examine provider-specific patterns of service use to identify the outliers from local or national norms. Further investigation would be necessary to determine if providers failed to follow practice standards without clear justification. Enforcement actions could include mandatory continuing education to improve adherence to standards or financial penalties for providers whose performance does not improve.

Federal programs (and private insurers) could present providers with a scorecard benchmarking their performance against the average provider performance in their market. Learning that they are outside professional norms could be a strong incentive for individual providers to improve their performance. In addition, AHRQ could direct resources for further study of methods to promote adherence to clinical standards.

CARE MANAGEMENT AND COORDINATION. Much of American health care is uncoordinated and inefficient, resulting in less than optimal care and higher costs.[38] Providers often do not share information that could reduce unnecessary services and avoid medical errors. Team approaches to patient care are uncommon in outpatient settings, and the patient's own role is often overlooked. Private and public health programs have started exploring ways to improve care coordination, including monitoring patient health status between visits and encouraging patient self-management.

Tightly managed health maintenance organizations (HMOs) might save 15 percent or more compared with plans that do not manage care.[39] Those potential savings led to growth of managed care plans during the 1990s, but such plans have proven unpopular with middle-class consumers.[40] Today, most people's plans offer little care coordination. Working-age people with employer-sponsored insurance primarily enroll in loosely managed preferred provider organizations, and most seniors are in traditional fee-for-service Medicare.

In contrast, Medicaid has long used managed care methods to control costs. Medicaid programs rely on direct management of health services to discourage unnecessary spending while maintaining reasonable access to care. During the 1990s Medicaid managed care grew rapidly as states used federal waivers to shift large numbers of beneficiaries out of fee-for-service programs.[41] By 2002, more than half of all Medicaid beneficiaries were enrolled in HMOs or primary care case management programs. Case management coordinates care across multiple providers, helping patients with complex health problems to obtain services at the lowest level of care that is medically appropriate.[42]

Many states also use disease management programs, which focus on specific diseases such as asthma, diabetes, high-risk pregnancies, and other conditions that account for substantial Medicaid spending. Although disease management programs vary considerably in their use of specific techniques, the programs have three common elements—they focus on the patient, providing education on managing their disease; they actively monitor the patient's condition and treatment protocols; and they coordinate care across providers, facilitating the sharing of information during the course of treatment.[43]

Medicare has several demonstration projects under way, and several completed projects, to test disease management approaches for patients with chronic conditions and complex health needs. Numerous interventions are being tried, including case management for high-cost beneficiaries, patient monitoring, data sharing, use of clinical guidelines, telemedicine, and patient support organizations.[44] However, more should be done to promote coordination between Medicare and Medicaid for low-income patients who often require a wide array of acute and long-term care services.

It is too early to determine whether disease management programs can reduce overall health spending.[45] Such programs incur additional costs for screening, monitoring, and educating patients, and it is unclear whether those costs are offset by savings from reduced use of other health services. More work is needed to determine the most effective combination of disease management tools and techniques for high-cost patients. When applied to a working population, disease management can also reduce absenteeism and increase work productivity.

One key to promoting coordinated care is financial incentives. Fee-for-service payments encourage physicians to see more patients for shorter office visits, and it is difficult to provide effective coordination in a fifteen-minute visit. Introducing a case manager, typically a nurse, reduces the demand on physician time but is resisted by some physicians as an imposition on their practice style. Alternatively, directly rewarding physician involvement could promote coordinated care. In addition, better patient management might be achieved if physicians were paid an additional amount for coordinating with case managers and other providers.

A variety of approaches should be tested to determine the optimal payment policy. P4P systems could include care coordination as one of the standards of performance. Medicare has experimented with a single bundled payment for hospital and physician services provided to cardiac patients and found that such an approach fosters efficiency. Recently, the CMS announced a gain-sharing project, in which hospitals would share with doctors some of the savings from joint efforts to improve care.[46]

END-OF-LIFE CARE. Because they cover the major health expenses of elderly Americans, Medicare and Medicaid bear much of the cost of dying in the United States, paying for about three-fourths of the total cost of care for seniors in their last year of life. About a quarter of total Medicare and Medicaid outlays is spent on care of patients in their last year of life, though such patients account for only 5 percent of the elderly population.[47]

Although many seniors prefer not to die in the hospital, inpatient hospital services account for more than 40 percent of the total paid by public and private insurance and out-of-pocket spending for seniors in their last year of life.[48] An alternative for some Medicare patients is hospice care, which provides palliative services (including skilled nursing care, medications for pain management, social services, short-term inpatient care, and other services) to those expected to live no more than six months. During the mid-1990s, hospice services accounted for only about 2 percent of total spending for seniors in their last year of life. The use of Medicare's hospice benefit has grown in recent years, with program outlays rising from $6.7 billion in 2004 to $9.8 billion in 2006.[49]

Much of the high cost of dying is from treating severe disease and functional impairment.[50] Greater adherence to evidence-based medical guidelines would help minimize unnecessary spending. Coordination between acute care and long-term care providers, and between Medicare and Medicaid, should also be improved. End-of-life care involves the full spectrum of acute- and long-term care services and financing streams that are not well coordinated today.

LOWER-COST DELIVERY SETTINGS. Visits to hospital emergency departments (EDs) increased 26 percent over the past decade, to about 114 million visits annually by 2003.[51] Close to one-third of those visits were classified as nonurgent or semi-urgent. Routine care in the ED is expensive, with charges estimated at two to five times higher than a typical office visit.[52]

A number of factors contribute to high ED use, including a growing uninsured population that is dependent on the ED for care. The Emergency Medical Treatment and Active Labor Act (EMTALA) of 1986 requires hospital EDs to screen all patients and stabilize them if necessary, regardless of their ability to pay.[53]

Many people with insurance coverage also use the ED for routine care. Medicaid patients are significantly more likely to use ED services than the uninsured or those with private coverage.[54] That may be due to their greater need for medical services, little or no cost sharing, and lower access to office-based physicians. Federal health insurance programs could encourage their beneficiaries to use lower-cost sites of care, perhaps by charging a fee to beneficiaries who habitually use the ED for routine care.[55] Other policies would improve access to lower-cost sites of care. For example, states might allow Medicaid patients to use walk-in health clinics operating in major retail chains, or federally financed health clinics might expand their hours to accommodate patients after most physician offices are closed.[56]

HEALTH PROMOTION AND DISEASE PREVENTION. The poor health habits of average Americans—smoking, inappropriate use of alcohol and drugs, poor diet, lack of exercise, and failure to seek timely help for illnesses—add significantly to the cost of health care in the United States. According to one analysis, 40 percent of deaths are the result of such poor health habits.[57] Chronic diseases, including diabetes, cancer, and cardiovascular diseases, account for 70 percent of deaths in the United States, and the cost of caring for people with these chronic diseases accounts for more than three-fourths of the nation's medical care costs.[58]

Although the concepts of health promotion and disease prevention have gained popularity among policymakers and the public, it is unclear whether such policies would yield substantial cost savings. A study published in 2000 found that increased participation in regular moderate exercise among the more than 88 million inactive adults might reduce national medical costs by as much as $77 billion annually, or almost 5 percent of national health expenditures.[59] However, wide-scale behavioral change is unlikely even with the most ambitious health promotion campaign.

The obesity "epidemic" illustrates this challenge. Almost one-third of the U.S. adult population is obese, and approximately two-thirds of adults are obese or overweight. Excess weight is a risk factor for type 2 diabetes, high blood pressure, coronary heart disease, stroke, and many types of cancer. Obese individuals are estimated to have inpatient and ambulatory care costs up to 36 percent higher than the general population.[60]

Much of this problem is preventable—poor diets and sedentary lifestyles are major contributors to obesity. However, despite widespread knowledge that proper diet and exercise can reduce the risk of expensive and debilitating disease, many people remain unwilling or unable to change their behavior. In some cases, environmental or social conditions compound the problem. For instance, lack of supermarkets in low-income areas and the pervasiveness of "supersize me" fast food restaurants offering cheap, high-calorie food make it more difficult to maintain healthy eating habits.

Some interventions, including childhood vaccination campaigns and smoking cessation programs, have been successful in preventing disease and generating cost savings. Researchers for the Centers for Disease Control and Prevention estimate that routine childhood immunizations reduce direct medical costs by $9.9 billion.[61] California estimates that its statewide tobacco prevention program resulted in overall cost savings of $8.4 billion between 1990 and 1998.[62] Nationwide, about 22 percent of adults are smokers today, compared with 33 percent in 1979.[63]

Greater use can be made of proven methods to reduce the cost of preventable disease. In particular, not all state Medicaid programs cover smoking cessation treatments even though smoking is more prevalent among low-income populations. In 2003 thirteen states did not cover such treatments despite the availability of funds earmarked for that purpose through the multistate tobacco settlement reached in 1998.[64]

Even successful health promotion and disease prevention activities may not reduce health care spending over the long term. Efforts that extend healthy life spans might only defer the need for expensive health care to later ages. Some interventions, such as medical screening, may not be cost-effective since a large number of people may be screened to identify the few who might have a disease, the screening and follow-up investigations and treatment can be expensive, and individuals incorrectly diagnosed as having the disease will incur both the cost and the physical consequences of unnecessary follow-up treatment.

Another impediment to better health is the failure of many people to adhere to their treatment regimens or to obtain care in an efficient manner. Recently, several state Medicaid programs have taken steps to encourage their enrollees to use health benefits more appropriately. West Virginia, for example, will offer enrollees enhanced coverage if they formally agree to take their medications, adhere to health improvement programs and health screening, not miss appointments, and use the hospital emergency room only for emergencies.[65] Those who choose the enhanced package will receive an array of preventive health services (including tobacco cessation, nutritional education, diabetes care, and chemical dependency/mental health services).

Promoting Consumerism and Competition

Numerous policy changes are required to introduce effective competition and informed consumer and provider decisionmaking into the health care market. Beyond prerequisites for effective market reform already discussed, such as payment methods that better reflect local market conditions, price transparency, and better information on the clinical effectiveness and quality of care, other possible steps include implementing premium support and related consumer-directed purchasing models and capping the exclusion of private health insurance premiums from taxable income.

PREMIUM SUPPORT. The Federal Employees Health Benefits Program is often cited as a model for the reform of Medicare and the broader health system. Under FEHBP, federal employees and retirees have a wide choice of competing health plans. About three-quarters of the insurance premium is paid by the government based on the average bid from the plans, with the remainder paid by enrollees.[66]

All plans in FEHBP are required to offer coverage for hospitalization, physician services, and other essential care, but they can augment the basic package of benefits. An enrollee willing to pay the extra premium may choose a health plan that is more expensive than average. This arrangement, often referred to as "premium support," limits the financial exposure of the federal government without unduly restricting consumers. It also fosters competition among the health plans, providing an incentive for the plans to manage their costs and improve their benefits as a way of gaining market share.

Several experts have proposed a premium support reform for Medicare.[67] The core of such a reform already exists in Medicare Advantage, which offers beneficiaries a choice of health plans as an alternative to traditional Medicare. Under full premium support, traditional Medicare would be placed on the same competitive footing as Medicare

Advantage plans, adjusting its premium and benefits to meet the competition from other plans.

Traditional Medicare would be given the same risk-adjusted subsidy for a beneficiary's care as the private plans receive. This is a controversial change from current practice. To be successful, traditional Medicare would need expanded authority to manage its costs, improve efficiency, and become a better purchaser of health services.

The Medicare Modernization Act (MMA) of 2003 used the premium support concept in designing the outpatient prescription drug benefit, which pays a subsidy based on the average premium offered by competing private plans. Narrowing competition to a single health benefit substantially reduces the scope for efficiency improvements, however, since the private drug plans cannot realize the potential savings from a well-managed pharmacy benefit that reduces use of inpatient and other services.

The MMA also included a voluntary test of premium support that would introduce direct price competition between traditional Medicare and Medicare Advantage plans. Scheduled to begin January 2010 in a limited number of local markets, the "Comparative Cost Adjustment Program" would charge a higher (or lower) Part B premium to enrollees in traditional Medicare if the cost of that program was higher (or lower) than the average cost of all plans in a market area. This would encourage enrollment in more efficient plans that charge lower premiums and put market pressure on both private plans and traditional Medicare to seek greater efficiency. The demonstration is unlikely to be implemented, however; previous attempts to test competitive pricing during the 1990s were halted because of opposition from health plans and local politicians.[68]

PREMIUM ASSISTANCE AND OTHER DEFINED CONTRIBUTION APPROACHES. Both Medicaid and SCHIP programs may provide premium assistance to beneficiaries who are offered insurance by an employer. Buying into an employer's health plan can be cost-effective, although states generally must supplement the private policies to ensure full coverage for services and to pay deductibles and copayments that are typically higher than allowed in Medicaid.[69]

The CMS introduced the Health Insurance Flexibility and Accountability (HIFA) initiative in 2001, which allows states to restructure their

Medicaid and SCHIP programs—including limiting enrollment, changing benefits, and increasing beneficiary cost sharing—and encourages the use of premium assistance.[70] The 2005 Deficit Reduction Act gave states even more flexibility to redesign their Medicaid programs, including the ability to customize benefits for different groups of beneficiaries.

Florida is implementing fundamental changes in its Medicaid program.[71] Instead of receiving a fixed set of benefits, enrollees will be given a fixed subsidy to meet their likely use of health services. The risk-adjusted premium can be used to enroll in a Medicaid managed care plan or to buy into an employer plan or individual coverage. Managed care plans will have new authority to determine the benefits they will provide. Adults, except for pregnant women, will be subject to a limit on the total cost of benefits allowed each year. Individuals who opt out of the Medicaid program by purchasing private insurance will receive no subsidies from the state other than their risk-adjusted premium.

There are a host of uncertainties associated with a reform as sweeping as Florida's.[72] Accurate risk adjustment is essential to ensure beneficiaries retain access to necessary care, but even the best estimation methods will have difficulty accurately predicting future use of services. Rising health costs may erode the beneficiary's purchasing power unless states raise subsidy levels over time. Medicaid beneficiaries will need assistance with their health plan choices, and most states are not equipped to provide that level of consumer protection.

States have implemented other reforms that provide Medicaid beneficiaries with individual budgets for care, giving them more control over how that money is spent. There is considerable interest among states in using this approach for the provision of personal care services.[73] Cash and Counseling gives Medicaid beneficiaries who are eligible for personal care services a consumer-directed allowance in lieu of traditional agency services. Beneficiaries (or their family caregivers) can choose the combination of goods and services that they prefer, including hiring a relative to provide assistance rather than relying on a home aide. This approach improved patient satisfaction without increasing program costs.[74] Twenty-two states have established or are actively planning programs for the frail elderly using this model, and the CMS has encouraged further state experimentation in this area.[75]

HEALTH SAVINGS ACCOUNTS. Congress authorized high-deductible insurance tied to tax-favored health savings accounts (HSA) in 2003, eliciting substantial interest among employers. Increasing the deductible makes beneficiaries more aware of the cost of their routine care and generally lowers the insurance premium. Many employers contribute a portion of the premium savings to the HSA, which helps their employees with the higher out-of-pocket cost.

The FEHBP introduced the option of high-deductible insurance coupled with HSAs for federal employees and retirees in 2005.[76] The new plans generally cover the same services as traditional FEHBP plans.[77] Enrollee deductibles are about twice as large as under traditional plans, but premiums are lower and contributions to the enrollee's HSA by the health plan are substantial. In 2005 enrollees in the three largest high-deductible plans saved an average of $90 a month for individual coverage and $200 a month for family coverage, compared with the average premium charged by traditional plans.

It is too early to assess the impact of high-deductible coverage on the use of services or the cost of the federal program. The new FEHBP plans provide online access to decision support tools that could help beneficiaries assess their treatment options. Information on cost and quality is limited, however, reflecting the paucity of such information in the health system as a whole. Enrollees in the new plans were younger and earned higher federal salaries than the average FEHBP enrollee, raising concerns that such plans might disproportionately attract younger and healthier people. Although risk selection could raise the cost of traditional plans, that is not an issue for the foreseeable future because enrollment in those plans is very low—7,500 out of a pool of 8 million federal employees, retirees, and family members.[78]

High-deductible health plans with a tax-favored savings account were first authorized for Medicare in 1997.[79] However, such plans have never been offered to beneficiaries. The CMS recently announced a new initiative to test more flexible approaches.[80] If employers adopt HSAs widely, future generations of seniors may want a similar option when they become eligible for Medicare.

TAX EXCLUSION. Reforming the tax treatment of health insurance would promote greater cost consciousness on the part of both consumers and providers. Capping or eliminating the tax exclusion for employer-sponsored insurance would also increase federal revenue. A gradual reduction in the value of this tax break would give the market a chance to accommodate the shift in demand toward less generous benefits and greater cost-sharing requirements.

A capped exclusion would tax employees on any contributions for health insurance or other tax-preferred health spending that exceeded some limit, such as the average premiums paid by employers. Allowing the cap to grow less rapidly than the growth in average premiums would phase in the restriction on the tax break over time. If a cap set at average employer contributions made in 2004 was not indexed, the Joint Committee on Taxation estimates that federal revenue would increase by about $700 billion between 2006 and 2015.[81]

A cap on the private insurance subsidy would initially increase the cost of coverage for high-income individuals, but eventually everyone would be affected. Loss of the tax subsidy would raise the cost of health coverage, encouraging the purchase of less generous policies. It could also cause some people to drop their coverage altogether. This reform is politically unpopular but holds great potential for health system reform.

Other Options

Beyond the considerable influence of the major health entitlement programs, other government entities contribute to the legal, institutional, and scientific structure in which public and private health programs operate. We focus on two policy options: improving the Food and Drug Administration's approval process for prescription drugs and restructuring the tort liability system to promote better quality of care.

DRUG APPROVALS. One of the many functions of the Food and Drug Administration is to protect consumers from unsafe or ineffective drugs while ensuring that the regulatory process does not unduly impede the introduction of innovative new products to the market.[82] This delicate balancing act has been the subject of intense public scrutiny after the FDA failed to detect rare but serious side effects that emerged with some popular medications, including increased risk of cardiovascular disease associated with the Cox-2 painkiller Vioxx.

The limited size and narrow focus of clinical trials in the drug approval process make them unlikely to identify problems that occur very rarely or arise because of interactions with other medical treatments or in patients with multiple conditions. Lengthening clinical trials would add to the cost of drug development without significantly adding to the safety of approved products.

Clinical trials typically measure the safety and effectiveness of a new drug against a placebo rather than against alternative therapies. Head-to-head trials of pharmaceuticals might yield insights about their comparative effectiveness. However, such trials would be substantially longer and more expensive. Drug approvals would be slowed significantly to the disadvantage of some patients who could benefit from a new treatment, but uncertainties about the benefits and risks of the new product would remain. This argues for paying greater attention to the health effects of new drugs once they are on the market.

The FDA is taking steps to beef up its postmarketing surveillance of new drugs.[83] Broader investment in health IT, including electronic medical records, would give the FDA real-time access to information on adverse events. New tools are being developed that would more rapidly detect a pattern of clinical results that needs investigation. Data collected under the Medicare drug benefit should also be used to identify safety problems.

Requiring labels that identify drugs as being in their first two years on the market would increase consumer awareness of their use of a newly approved therapy, which could prompt patients to report possible adverse effects to their physicians.[84] An advertising ban during that period would reduce consumer demand for new drugs and slow their diffusion into medical practice. This would give the FDA more time to deal with any safety issues that arise, but it would also delay some patients' access to the therapeutic benefits of the new drug.

A slowdown in drug approvals has raised concerns about the complexity and adequacy of the approval process. In 2005 the FDA approved twenty new drugs, down from thirty-six in 2004.[85] The development and review process is not keeping pace with drug discovery, to a great extent because scientists test new discoveries using inefficient tools and techniques.

The FDA's Critical Path Initiative is an effort to modernize the process through which basic scientific discoveries translate into new medical treatments.[86] By implementing standards for clinical trial design and uniform statistical methodologies, early warnings could predict failure before advanced clinical trials take place. Helping pharmaceutical companies "fail faster" on drugs that eventually would not be approved could significantly reduce the cost of drug development. For example, shifting 5 percent of clinical failures from Phase III to Phase I trials would reduce costs by $15 million to $20 million.[87] In addition, clearer guidance for product approvals and better communication between FDA and pharmaceutical companies can smooth the development process and reduce the cost of multiple reviews by the agency.

The FDA can promote price competition in the drug market by introducing close substitutes for brand name products more quickly. Some of that competition comes from other brand name drugs in a therapeutic class, the "me-too" drugs that are different molecules designed to treat a common disease. Even stronger price pressure is exerted by the entry of generic drugs. Generic drugs have the same active ingredients as the brand name version, and usually cost 60 to 90 percent less.[88] The price drops the most with the first generic alternative to a brand-name drug and continues to fall as each new competitor reaches the market.

With many blockbuster drugs going off patent, the FDA faces a growing backlog of applications to bring new generic products to the market. The strong demand for lower-cost pharmaceuticals has attracted competition within the generic market, resulting in multiple applications to sell generic versions of many drugs. To manage the backlog, the FDA gives priority to the first application for a generic equivalent of a branded product. Better funding for the FDA's Office of Generic Drug Approval, perhaps through user fees levied on the manufacturers, could speed the approval process.

Brand-name manufacturers have used a variety of techniques to reduce generic competition, such as paying generic manufacturers to stay out of the market.[89] Brand manufacturers also may threaten to launch their own authorized generics, reducing the market share available to generic manufacturers. The Federal Trade Commission is investigating actions that could limit these techniques.

Biologics—complex molecules, such as proteins, derived from living organisms and used as medical treatments—represent a significant part of the U.S. drug industry, with sales expected to top $57 billion by 2010.[90] The FDA approval process for biologics is complicated because their manufacture involves living organisms. The Hatch-Waxman Act provides a clear path for approval of generic drugs, but not for generic, or "follow-on," biologics.[91] Moreover, there are difficult scientific questions about what constitutes bioequivalence for these products. Consequently, the potential for price-reducing competition in the biologics market is sharply attenuated.

MALPRACTICE REFORM. The medical liability insurance system is in upheaval, with rapid increases in insurance premiums and the exit of major insurance carriers from the medical liability market. Between 2000 and 2002, malpractice insurance premiums rose by 15 percent on average for all physicians.[92] High-risk specialties faced even larger premium hikes: 22 percent for obstetricians-gynecologists and 33 percent for internists and general surgeons. A general surgeon in Miami could expect to pay at least $174,000 a year for liability coverage in 2002.[93]

As premiums rose, the availability of malpractice insurance diminished. The St. Paul Companies, which was the largest malpractice insurer during the 1990s, dropped out of that market in 2002.[94] Other large insurance carriers have also exited the market.

These problems and heightened public awareness of patient safety problems have prompted a feverish debate over capping malpractice awards and attorneys' fees. Physicians and liability insurers argue that such caps would slow the growth of malpractice premiums and reduce overall health spending. Trial lawyers argue that this unfairly penalizes patients who have suffered from a medical mistake and have no other recourse.

Capping malpractice awards would lower the cost of malpractice insurance, but the impact on overall health costs would be modest. California was one of the earliest states to impose such a cap through the Medical Injury Compensation Reform Act (MICRA) of 1975, which restricts noneconomic damages to $250,000 and limits attorneys' fees.[95] Federal legislation modeled after MICRA would lower malpractice premiums by 25 to 30 percent.[96] However, malpractice premiums amount to less than 2 percent of overall health spending, resulting in only a 0.5 percent reduction in national health expenditures.

Additional savings are possible from reducing "defensive medicine," where physicians use tests and procedures that have little therapeutic value but that provide a legal defense against a malpractice claim. The adoption of caps on awards reduced spending for heart disease and heart attack patients by about 4 percent with no adverse effect on mortality rates or complications.[97] However, the Congressional Budget Office (CBO) found no evidence that tort reforms reduced medical spending when considering a broader set of ailments.[98]

Tort reform could be part of a broader effort to improve patient safety and provide appropriate redress for injured patients. More attention should be placed on preventing medical errors. Reengineering medical workplaces can make errors less common and improve the response of the system when errors do occur.[99] Focusing blame on those involved with an error is a poor strategy for improving patient safety, as most errors are the result of mistakes by competent people working in stressful situations. More could be done to improve provider performance through training, guidelines, performance measurement, and research on patient safety.

When an injury does occur, patients need better access to a fairer liability system. Few patients who have experienced medical negligence bring lawsuits, and few receive compensation.[100] Claims are resolved slowly, on average four to five years from the date of an incident.[101] Injured patients receive only about 40 percent of the malpractice insurance payments, with the rest going to legal and administrative fees. Awards can be inequitable. Many patients with meritorious claims receive nothing, while others are granted judgments that seem disproportionate to the severity of their injury.

More structured payment rules and the use of alternative methods for resolving malpractice claims would make the system more equitable. One proposal would tie disclosure of the circumstances of patient injury with an offer to pay for out-of-pocket losses in exchange for an agreement not to pursue claims for pain and suffering.[102] Other proposals include automatic payment for avoidable events that are identified in advance, replacing the tort liability system with an administrative compensation system (similar to workers compensation), and the creation of specialized health courts that could be more systematic in their evaluation of malpractice cases.[103]

Capping Health Spending

Even if an efficient health system can be achieved, that does not dictate either the level of health spending or its rate of growth. Consequently, policymakers must consider whether to limit directly the growth of health spending. Spending limits take the regulatory approach, which tends to favor social judgments over individual preferences, to an extreme. As a society, we have never directly confronted the question of how much, in a resource-constrained world, we are individually and collectively willing to devote to health care, and how much to all other goods and services. However, there have been sporadic attempts to limit spending in Medicaid and Medicare.

During the mid-1990s, the Oregon Health Plan expanded Medicaid coverage to most low-income residents. To hold down budgetary costs, the state prioritized health care services based on their clinical effectiveness as judged by medical experts and reviewed through a series of town meetings. This process was intended to establish both a scientific basis and a community standard for acceptable care, bringing the public's views regarding adequate care to bear on the budget process. The goal was to pay for the most appropriate care for each patient. The experiment has not continued, however. Fiscal pressures and a slowing state economy essentially halted the project by 2003, with the Oregon Health Plan reverting to a more traditional Medicaid program.[104]

Congress imposed several methods of limiting the growth of Medicare payments for physician services during the 1990s. The current formula, called the sustainable growth rate (SGR), ties physician spending to growth in the economy. Medicare adjusts its physician payment rates annually to allow for increases in the cost of providing care. If Medicare physician outlays grow faster than the SGR, the annual update is reduced. That lowers the *prices* paid for physician services across the board to account for excess growth in *expenditures,* which reflect increases in the volume and complexity of services as well as price increases.

The SGR has generated a difficult political problem for Congress. Medicare physician spending, like other health costs, is growing more rapidly than GDP (gross domestic product). As a result, the formula automatically imposes 4 to 5 percent reductions in Medicare's payment rates virtually every year for the foreseeable future. Fee reductions of this magnitude are untenable and, if sustained, would reduce access to care as doctors take fewer Medicare patients in favor of more lucrative business.

However, permanently restoring the payment reductions would cost several hundred billion dollars over the next decade. Any payment relief granted to physicians also increases beneficiary premiums for Medicare Part B, which are set at 25 percent of program costs. As a result, policymakers have resorted to one-year fixes, deferring the fee reduction and providing a small increase in most years rather than establishing a new permanent payment policy.

The SGR illustrates the challenges of broad efforts to cap the growth of health spending. Without great care in their application, the government's budgetary savings might result in less access to necessary care or higher private spending without substantially lowering the growth of overall health spending.[105] Any limitation on spending will ultimately entail difficult choices about what care is to be delivered to whom under what circumstances. Such decisions might be made through a political process, but they might also be made by consumers facing higher out-of-pocket expenses for their care.

Conclusion

A plethora of policy options is available that could help ameliorate the federal health spending crisis. Many of those options are likely to produce one-time savings rather than a permanent reduction in the growth of outlays—not an ideal solution to the fiscal problem, but one that at least buys time for further policy innovation. Every option requires development and testing to be implemented in a way that balances reducing costs, ensuring access to care, promoting high quality, and other objectives. Society does not lack ideas to test, but it may lack the political will to proceed.

This volume focuses on the major federal programs that finance the cost of health care through insurance or the direct provision of services. Medicare and Medicaid are the largest of those programs, and both face immediate financing problems that will only worsen with the aging baby boom generation and the continuing trend toward the use of more services and greater complexity of care. Other programs (SCHIP, VHA, and

TRICARE) are smaller and pose less of a fiscal threat, but they are also subject to rising cost pressures.

The succeeding chapters explore in greater depth the performance of those programs and the steps that could be taken to improve their efficiency, better serve their beneficiary populations, and slow their spending growth. Lessons from such policy initiatives can help policymakers—and society as a whole—work toward a high-value health system.

Notes

1. Medicare provides coverage to persons under age 65 who receive payments under Social Security's Disability Insurance program, but only after a 24-month waiting period.

2. Mark V. Pauly, "The Economics of Moral Hazard," *American Economic Review* 58, no. 3, pt. I (1968): 531–37.

3. Amy Finkelstein, "The Aggregate Effects of Health Insurance: Evidence from the Introduction of Medicare," Working Paper (Cambridge, Mass.: National Bureau of Economic Research, April 2006); *Quarterly Journal of Economics* (February 2007, forthcoming).

4. Personal communication with John Sheils, February 2, 2006. The estimating methodology is described in John Sheils and Randall Haught, "The Cost of Tax-Exempt Health Benefits in 2004," *Health Affairs* web exclusive, February 25, 2004: W4-106–W4-112 (http://content.healthaffairs.org/cgi/content/full/hlthaff.w4.106v1/DC1).

5. Other tax preferences include the deduction for out-of-pocket health spending exceeding 7.5 percent of adjusted gross income, tax preferences for contributions to medical savings accounts or health savings accounts, and the exclusion of premiums from the incomes of the self-employed.

6. Leonard E. Burman and Amelia Gruber, "First, Do No Harm: Designing Tax Incentives for Health Insurance," *National Tax Journal* 54, no. 3 (September 2001): 473–93.

7. John E. Wennberg, Elliot S. Fisher, and Jonathan S. Skinner, "Geography and the Debate over Medicare Reform," *Health Affairs* web exclusive, February 13, 2002: W2-96–W2-114 (http://content.healthaffairs.org/cgi/content/full/hlthaff.w2.96v1/DC1).

8. Dartmouth Atlas of Health Care, *The Care of Patients with Severe Chronic Illness* (Hanover, NH: Center for the Evaluative Clinical Sciences, Dartmouth Medical School, 2006) (http://www.dartmouthatlas.org/atlases/2006_Chronic_Care_Atlas.pdf).

9. Elliott S. Fisher and others, "The Implications of Regional Variations in Medicare Spending. Part 2: Health Outcomes and Satisfaction with Care," *Annals of Internal Medicine* 138, no. 4 (February 18, 2003): 288–98.

10. Earl P. Steinberg and Bryan R. Luce, "Evidence Based? Caveat Emptor!" *Health Affairs* 24 (January/February 2005): 80–92. See also David M. Eddy, "Evidence-Based Medicine: A Unified Approach," *Health Affairs* 24 (January-February 2005): 9–17.

11. Eddy, "Evidence-Based Medicine."

12. The U.S. Census Bureau reports that 46.6 million people, or 15.9 percent of the population, were uninsured for all of 2005; see Carmen DeNavas-Walt, Bernadette D. Proctor, and Cheryl Hill Lee, "Income, Poverty, and Health Insurance Coverage in the United States: 2005," *Current Population Reports,* P60-231 (Government Printing Office, 2006). Many analysts believe that the Census estimate is closer to the number of uninsured at a specific point in time during the year and that the number without insurance for the entire year is smaller. Panel surveys show that the number of uninsured at any time during the year is substantially larger than the Census estimate. See Congressional Budget Office (CBO), *How Many People Lack Health Insurance and For How Long?* (GPO, May 2003).

13. CBO, *How Many People Lack Health Insurance and For How Long?*

14. Jack Hadley and John Holahan, "Covering the Uninsured: How Much Would It Cost?" *Health Affairs* web exclusive, June 4, 2003: W3-250–W3-265 (http://content.healthaffairs.org/cgi/content/full/hlthaff.w3.250v1/DC1).

15. Lola Butcher, "Plans Put Provider Prices Out for Their Enrollees to Inspect," *Managed Care* 15, no. 2 (February 2006) (managedcaremag.com/archives/0602/0602.consumer.html).

16. Mary Agnes Carey, "Bush Expected To Discuss Price Transparency at AHA Meeting," *CQ Healthbeat News,* April 27, 2006.

17. Cathy Schoen and others, "Insured but Not Protected: How Many Adults Are Underinsured?" *Health Affairs* web exclusive, June 14, 2005: W5-289–W5-302 (http://content.healthaffairs.org/cgi/content/full/hlthaff.w5.289/DC1).

18. Alan C. Monheit, "Persistence in Health Expenditures: Prevalence and Consequences," *Medical Care* 41 (July 2003 Supplement): III-53–III-64.

19. Karen Davis, "Consumer-Directed Health Care: Will It Improve Health System Performance?" *Health Services Research* 39 (August 2004, Part II): 1219–33.

20. This list is based on John F. Cogan, R. Glenn Hubbard, and Daniel P. Kessler, *Healthy, Wealthy, and Wise: Five Steps to a Better Health Care System* (Washington: AEI Press, 2005; Stanford, Calif.: Hoover Institution, 2005).

21. Cristina Boccuti and Marilyn Moon, "Comparing Medicare and Private Insurers: Growth Rates in Spending over Three Decades," *Health Affairs* 22 (March/April 2003): 230–37.

22. Michael J. O'Grady, "Health Insurance Spending Growth—How Does Medicare Compare?" Joint Economic Committee, U.S. Congress (GPO, June 10, 2003).

23. Sandra Christensen, "Volume Response to Exogenous Changes in Medicare's Payment Policies," *Health Services Research* 27, no. 1 (April 1992): 65–79.

24. Joseph R. Antos, "Is There a Right Way to Promote Health Insurance through the Tax System?" *National Tax Journal* LIX, no. 3 (September 2006): 477-490. See also President's Advisory Panel on Federal Tax Reform, *Simple, Fair, and Pro-Growth: Proposals to Fix America's Tax System* (November 2005) (www.taxreformpanel.gov/final-report/).

25. Medicare's PPS system is not purely diagnosis based. Physicians often face an array of possible diagnoses with different prices and have an incentive to treat more intensively to justify a higher price.

26. Karen Milgate and Sharon Bee Cheng, "Pay-For-Performance: The Med-PAC Perspective," *Health Affairs* 25 (March-April 2006): 413–19.

27. Michael F. Cannon, "Pay-for-Performance: Is Medicare a Good Candidate," Cato Institute Working Paper (www.cato.org/pub_display.php?pub_id= 6557); *Yale Journal of Health Policy, Law, and Ethics* (2007, forthcoming).

28. Cindy Skrzycki, "Bidding to Equip Medicare," *Washington Post*, May 2, 2006, p. D1.

29. CBO, *Prices for Brand-Name Drugs Under Selected Federal Programs* (GPO, June 2005) p. 4.

30. Office of the National Coordinator for Health Information Technology, U.S. Department of Health and Human Services, *Directory of Federal HIT Programs*, 2006 (www.hhs.gov/healthit/federalprojectlist.html#initiativestable).

31. George W. Bush. "Executive Order: Promoting Quality and Efficient Health Care in Federal Government Administered or Sponsored Health Care Programs," August 22, 2006 (www.whitehouse.gov/news/releases/2006/08/2006 0822-2.html).

32. Centers for Medicare & Medicaid Services (CMS), "Fact Sheet: Physician Self-Referral Exceptions For Electronic Prescribing and Electronic Health Records Technology," August 1, 2006 (www.cms.hhs.gov/apps/media/press/release.asp? Counter=1920).

33. U.S. Government Accountability Office (GAO), *Domestic and Offshore Outsourcing of Personal Information in Medicare, Medicaid, and TRICARE,* GAO-06-676 (September 6, 2006).

34. U.S. Department of Health and Human Services (HHS), "Medicare Posts Hospital Payment Information," press release, June 1, 2006 (www.hhs.gov/news/ press/2006pres/20060601a.html).

35. The challenges of using clinical- and cost-effectiveness analysis in Medicare are discussed in Medicare Payment Advisory Commission (MedPAC), *Report to Congress: Issues in a Modernized Medicare Program,* June 2005.

36. Chris Ham, "Retracing the Oregon Trail: The Experience of Rationing and the Oregon Health Plan," *British Medical Journal* 316 (June 27, 1998): 1965–69.

37. CMS, *Medicare News: Medicare Revises Guidance For National Coverage Determinations with Evidence Development,* July 12, 2006 (www.cms. hhs.gov/apps/media/press/release.asp?Counter=1897). See also Barry M. Straube, "How Changes in the Medicare Coverage Process Have Facilitated the Spread of New Technologies," *Health Affairs* web exclusive, June 23, 2005: W5-314–W5-316 (http://content.healthaffairs.org/cgi/content/full/hlthaff. w5.314/DC1).

38. The need for care coordination in a Medicare context is discussed in Med-PAC, *Report to Congress: Increasing the Value of Medicare* (June 2006).

39. Verdon S. Staines, "Potential Impact of Managed Care on National Health Spending," *Health Affairs* 12 (Supplement 1993): 248–57.

40. Debra A. Draper and others, "The Changing Face of Managed Care," *Health Affairs* 21 (January/February 2002): 11–23.

41. Debra A. Draper, Robert E. Hurley, and Ashley C. Short, "Medicaid Managed Care: The Last Bastion of the HMO?" *Health Affairs* 23 (March/April 2004): 155–67.

42. Sandra M. Foote, "Population-Based Disease Management under Fee-For-Service Medicare," *Health Affairs* web exclusive, July 30, 2003: W3-342–W3-356 (http://content.healthaffairs.org/cgi/content/full/hlthaff.w3.342v1/DC1).

43. CBO, *High-Cost Medicare Beneficiaries* (GPO, May 2005).

44. MedPAC, *Report to Congress: Increasing the Value of Medicare*. See also Nora Super, *Medicare's Chronic Care Improvement Pilot Program: What Is Its Potential?* Issue Brief 797 (Washington: National Health Policy Forum, 2004); and Foote, "Population-Based Disease Management."

45. CBO, "An Analysis of the Literature on Disease Management Programs," letter to the Honorable Don Nickles, Senate Committee on the Budget, 108th Cong., 2d. sess., October 13, 2004 (www.cbo.gov/publications/bysubject.cfm?cat=9). See also Bruce Fireman, Joan Bartlett, and Joe Selby, "Can Disease Management Reduce Health Care Costs by Improving Quality?" *Health Affairs* 23 (November-December 2004): 63–75.

46. CMS, "CMS News: CMS Demonstration Program Supports Physician-Hospital Collaborations to Improve Quality of Care While Getting Better Value," September 6, 2006 (www.cms.hhs.gov/apps/media/press/release.asp?Counter=1957).

47. Donald R. Hoover and others, "Medical Expenditures during the Last Year of Life: Findings from the 1992–1996 Medicare Current Beneficiary Survey—Cost of Care," *Health Services Research* 37 (December 2002): 1625–642.

48. Ibid.

49. MedPAC, *Report to Congress: Increasing the Value of Medicare*.

50. Christopher Hogan and others, "Medicare Beneficiaries' Costs of Care in the Last Year of Life," *Health Affairs* 20 (July-August 2001): 188–95.

51. Peter J. Cunningham, "Medicaid/SCHIP Cuts and Hospital Emergency Department Use," *Health Affairs* 25 (January-February 2006): 237–47.

52. Institute of Medicine, *Hospital-Based Emergency Care: At the Breaking Point* (Washington, 2006).

53. Bruce Siegel, "The Emergency Department: Rethinking the Safety Net for the Safety Net," *Health Affairs* web exclusive, March 24, 2004: W4-146–W4-148 (http://content.healthaffairs.org/cgi/content/full/hlthaff.w4.146v1/DC1).

54. Cunningham, "Medicaid/SCHIP Cuts."

55. Such a fee in Medicare would be considered a penalty, not part of cost-sharing. Consequently, supplementary insurance (such as Medigap) would not cover the fee, which would be paid directly out of pocket by the beneficiary.

56. The growth of walk-in health clinics is assessed by Mary Kate Scott in *Health Care in the Express Lane: The Emergence of Retail Clinics* (Oakland, Calif.: California Healthcare Foundation, July 2006).

57. J. Michael McGinnis, Pamela Williams-Russo, and James R. Knickman, "The Case For More Active Policy Attention to Health Promotion," *Health Affairs* 21 (March-April 2002): 78–93. See also J. Michael McGinnis and William H. Foege, "Actual Causes of Death in the United States," *Journal of the American Medical Association* 270, no. 18 (1993): 2207–12.

58. HHS, "Prevention Makes Common 'Cents,'" September 2003 (aspe.hhs.gov/health/prevention/).

59. Michael Pratt, Caroline A. Macera, and Guijing Wang, "Higher Direct Medical Costs Associated with Physical Inactivity," *Physician and Sportsmedicine* 28, no. 10 (October 2000) (www.physsportsmed.com/issues/2000/10_00/pratt.htm).

60. HHS, "Prevention Makes Common 'Cents.'"

61. Fangjun Zhou and others, "Economic Evaluation of the 7-Vaccine Routine Child Immunization Schedule in the United States, 2001," *Pediatrics and Adolescent Medicine* 12 (December 2005): 1136–44.

62. HHS, "Prevention Makes Common 'Cents.'"

63. Kenneth E. Thorpe, "The Rise in Health Care Spending and What to Do about It," *Health Affairs* 24 (November-December 2005): 1436–445.

64. Helen A. Halpin, Nicole M. Bellows, and Sara B. McMenamin, "Medicaid Coverage For Tobacco-Dependence Treatments," *Health Affairs* 25 (March-April 2006): 550–56. In 2005 five states and the District of Columbia committed no tobacco settlement or tobacco tax money for tobacco prevention programs; see Campaign for Tobacco-Free Kids, *A Broken Promise to Our Children: The 1998 State Tobacco Settlement Seven Years Later*, November 30, 2005 (www.tobaccofreekids.org/reports/settlements/2006/fullreport.pdf).

65. Kaiser Commission on Medicaid and the Uninsured, "West Virginia Medicaid State Plan Amendment: Key Program Changes and Questions," July 2006 (www.kff.org/medicaid/7529.cfm).

66. The federal payment is equal to 72 percent of the average premium offered by the plans, weighted by enrollment. That payment is limited and cannot exceed 75 percent of the premium for any particular plan. See Karl Polzer, *The Federal Employees Health Benefits Program: What Lessons Can It Offer Policymakers,* Issue Brief 715 (Washington: National Health Policy Forum, March 12, 1998) (www.nhpf.org/pdfs_ib/IB715_FEHBP_3-12-98.pdf).

67. Henry J. Aaron and Robert D. Reischauer, "The Medicare Reform Debate: What Is the Next Step?" *Health Affairs* 14 (Winter 1995): 8–30; see also Gail R. Wilensky and Joseph P. Newhouse, "Medicare: What's Right? What's Wrong? What's Next?" *Health Affairs* 18 (January-February 1999): 92–106; and John Breaux and Bill Thomas, *Final Breaux-Thomas Medicare Reform Proposal* (Washington: National Bipartisan Commission on the Future of Medicare, 1999) (http://rs9.loc.gov/medicare/bbmt3159.html).

68. Len M. Nichols and Robert D. Reischauer, "Who Really Wants Price Competition in Medicare Managed Care?" *Health Affairs* 19 (September-October 2000): 30–43. See also Bryan Down, Robert Coulam, and Roger Feldman, "A Tale of Four Cities: Medicare Reform and Competitive Pricing," *Health Affairs* 19 (September-October 2000): 9–29.

69. Cynthia Shirk and Jennifer Ryan, "Premium Assistance in Medicaid and SCHIP: Ace in the Hole or House of Cards?" Issue Brief 812 (Washington: National Health Policy Forum, July 17, 2006) (www.nhpf.org/pdfs_ib/IB812_PremiumAssist_07-17-06.pdf?search=%22schip%20Medicaid%20%22 premium%20assistance%22%22).

70. Teresa A. Coughlin and others, "An Early Look at Ten State HIFA Medicaid Waivers," *Health Affairs* web exclusive, April 25, 2006: W204–W216 (http://content.healthaffairs.org/cgi/content/full/25/3/w204).

71. Kaiser Commission on Medicaid and the Uninsured, "Florida Medicaid Waiver: Key Program Changes and Issues," December 2005 (www.kff.org/medicaid/upload/7443.pdf).

72. Charles Milligan, Cynthia Woodcock, and Alice Burton, "Turning Medicaid Beneficiaries into Purchasers of Health Care: Critical Success Factors for Medicaid Consumer-Directed Health Purchasing," Issue Brief—State Coverage Initiatives (Washington: AcademyHealth, August 2006) (www.academyhealth.org/publications/briefs.htm).

73. Brenda C. Spillman, Kirsten J. Black, and Barbara A. Ormond, *Beyond Cash and Counseling: An Inventory of Individual Budget-Based Community Long-Term Care Programs for the Elderly,* Report 7485 (Menlo Park, Calif.: Kaiser Family Foundation, April 2006) (www.kff.org/medicaid/upload/7485.pdf).

74. Leslie Foster and others, "Improving the Quality of Medicaid Personal Assistance through Consumer Direction," *Health Affairs* web exclusive, March 26, 2003: W3-162–W3-175 (http://content.healthaffairs.org/cgi/content/full/hlthaff.w3.162v1/DC1); see also Stacy Dale and others, "The Effects of Cash and Counseling on Personal Care Services and Medicaid Costs in Arkansas," *Health Affairs* web exclusive, November 19, 2003: W3-566–W3-575 (http://content.healthaffairs.org/cgi/content/full/hlthaff.w3.566v1/DC1).

75. Spillman, Black, and Ormond, *Beyond Cash and Counseling.*

76. Other types of health accounts, including flexible savings accounts (FSAs) and health reimbursement arrangements (HRAs), are available through FEHBP and many private employers; see Office of Personnel Management, *Federal Employee Health Benefit Program: 2006 Plan Guide (RI 70-1 For Federal Civilian Employees),* 2006 (http://opm.gov/insure/06/guides/70-01). Such accounts provide tax breaks for out-of-pocket health spending but are not tied to high-deductible insurance. FSAs have a "use it or lose it" feature, requiring that any contributions to the account revert to the employer if they are not used by the end of the year. HRA balances may carry over from year to year, but they are not owned by the employee and are thus not portable in the event of a job change.

77. GAO, *Federal Employees Health Benefits Program: First-Year Experience with High-Deductible Health Plans and Health Savings Accounts,* GAO-06-271 (January 2006) (www.gao.gov/new.items/d06271.pdf).

78. Ibid.

79. The Balanced Budget Act of 1997 expanded the types of plans that could participate in what is now called Medicare Advantage, including preferred provider organizations, private fee-for-service plans, and medical savings accounts

(MSAs). MSAs are still authorized but have not been offered by any plan participating in Medicare Advantage.

80. CMS, "Medicare News: CMS Announces Steps to Improve Access to Consumer-Directed Health Plans in Medicare," July 10, 2006 (www.cms.hhs. gov/apps/media/press/release.asp?Counter=1894).

81. CBO, *Budget Options* (GPO, June 2005).

82. The Food and Drug Administration's mission is to ensure the safety, efficacy, and security of drugs, biological products, and medical devices, as well as the nation's food supply and cosmetics; see FDA, *FDA's Mission Statement,* undated (www.fda.gov/opacom/morechoices/mission.html). The FDA is also responsible for helping to speed innovations that make medicines and foods more effective, safer, and more affordable, and helping the public obtain accurate information on the medicines and foods they use.

83. Scott Gottlieb, "Opening Pandora's Pillbox: Using Modern Information Tools to Improve Drug Safety," *Health Affairs* 24 (July-August 2005): 938–48.

84. Institute of Medicine, *The Future of Drug Safety: Promoting and Protecting the Health of the Public* (Washington, 2006).

85. Pitts, "Trouble in the FDA Pipeline?" *Adverse Event Reporting News* 3, no. 6 (March 20, 2006): 3–5 (www.cmpi.org/viewstddoccontent.asp?detailid= 21&contenttypeid=2).

86. Food and Drug Administration, *Critical Path Initiative Fact Sheet,* undated (www.fda.gov/oc/initiatives/criticalpath/factsheet.html).

87. Pitts, "Trouble in the FDA Pipeline?"

88. Marc Kaufman, "Generic Drugs Hit Backlog at FDA," *Washington Post,* February 4, 2006, p. A1.

89. Bureau of National Affairs (BNA), "Brand-Name Drug Firms Resuming Payments to Keep Generics Out of Market, FTC Reports," *Pharmaceutical Law & Industry Report* 4, no.17 (April 28, 2006) (http://healthcenter.bna.com/ pic2/hc.nsf/id/BNAP-6PALR3?OpenDocument).

90. Bruce S. Manheim Jr., Patricia Granahan, and Kenneth J. Dow, "'Follow-On Biologics': Ensuring Continued Innovation in the Biotechnology Industry," *Health Affairs* 25 (March-April 2006): 394–404.

91. Henry Grabowski, Iain Cockburn, and Genia Long, "The Market for Follow-On Biologics: How Will It Evolve?" *Health Affairs* 25 (September-October 2006): 1291–1301.

92. CBO, "Limiting Tort Liability for Medical Malpractice," Economic & Budget Issue Brief, January 8, 2004.

93. Randall R. Bovbjerg and Robert Berenson, *Surmounting Myths and Mindsets in Medical Malpractice,* Health Policy Brief (Washington: Urban Institute, October 2005) (www.urban.org/UploadedPDF/411227_medical_malpractice.pdf).

94. Kenneth Thorpe, "The Medical Malpractice Crisis," *Health Affairs* web exclusive, January 21, 2004: W4-20–W4-30 (http://content.healthaffairs.org/cgi/ content/full/hlthaff.w4.20v1/DC1).

95. RAND Corporation, *Changing the Medical Malpractice Dispute Process: What Have We Learned from California's MICRA?* Research Brief (Santa Monica, Calif., 2004) (www.rand.org/pubs/research_briefs/RB9071/RB9071.pdf).

96. CBO, *Limiting Tort Liability for Medical Malpractice.*

97. Daniel P. Kessler and Mark B. McClellan, "Do Doctors Practice Defensive Medicine?" *Quarterly Journal of Economics* 111, no. 2 (1996): 353–90.

98. CBO, *The Effects of Tort Reform: Evidence from the States* (GPO, June 2004).

99. Bovbjerg and Berenson, *Surmounting Myths and Mindsets.*

100. Ibid.

101. Michelle M. Mello, *Understanding Medical Malpractice Insurance: A Primer,* Research Synthesis Report 8 (Princeton, N.J.: Robert Wood Johnson Foundation, January 2006) (www.rwjf.org/publications/synthesis/reports_and_ briefs/pdf/no10_primer.pdf#search=%22mello%20malpractice%20synthesis%22).

102. Bovbjerg and Berenson, *Surmounting Myths and Mindsets.*

103. Catherine T. Struve, "Improving the Medical Malpractice Litigation Process," *Health Affairs* 23 (July-August 2004): 33–41.

104. Wayne J. Guglielmo, "Why Oregon's Rationing Plan Is Gasping for Air," *Medical Economics,* October 8, 2004 (www.memag.com/memag/article/articleDetail.jsp?id=127172&pageID=1).

105. One could argue that government policy should not limit private health spending, which reflects the judgment of individuals about the value of the services and their willingness to pay. However, much of private health spending is financed through insurance, which is subsidized through the tax system. As Butler points out in a later chapter, society has a valid interest in the way publicly subsidized private funds are spent for health services.

3

The Challenge of Medicare

GAIL R. WILENSKY

T he Medicare program is central to efforts to slow the rate of growth of health care spending. As discussed in chapter 1, the rate at which Medicare grows (along with Medicaid) will largely determine how fast total federal spending grows in the future and how prodigious an effort is required to keep the federal deficit under control. At the same time, as I shall discuss in this chapter, it is politically unlikely that the growth of Medicare spending will be allowed to fall behind the growth in total health care spending. Hence, the future growth in Medicare spending will attest to the success or failure of efforts to moderate the growth of total health spending.

Background on Medicare

The Medicare program was enacted in 1965 with the objective of providing seniors with health care that would be comparable to the health

The author is a senior fellow at Project HOPE and would like to thank Michelle Fischer for her able assistance in researching and editing this chapter. Fischer, currently a major in the U.S. Army, Brooke Army Medical Center, Fort Sam Houston, served as the author's intern while she was a graduate student at George Washington University.

care available to the rest of the American population. Although most ana-lysts believe that Medicare has succeeded in fulfilling this basic objective, there are important differences between Medicare and the health care available to the privately insured population in coverage and organiza-tional structure of the delivery system.

Medicare as a Health Care Program

Medicare has four basic components. Part A, the Hospital Insurance pro-gram, covers inpatient hospital care and some home care, skilled nursing home care, and hospice care. It is financed by a portion of the Social Secu-rity wage tax—a 2.9 percent combined tax on employer and employee, although unlike the rest of the Social Security tax, the Medicare portion applies to all earned income. Part B, the Supplementary Medical Insur-ance program, covers outpatient hospital services, the remaining home health services, physician services, other services such as laboratory and diagnostic tests and durable medical equipment. Part C, also called Medicare Advantage, gives Medicare beneficiaries the option of enrolling in private plans—with at least the coverage of Parts A and B—that are paid on a capitated basis. Part D, which began in 2006, covers outpatient prescription drugs that are provided by private drug plans. The federal government contributions for Parts B and D come from general revenue. Medicare beneficiaries pay part of the cost of both Part B and Part D with premiums.

The Medicare benefit package contains more home care coverage than most plans for the under-65 population and, although limited, some nurs-ing home coverage. However, except for the catastrophic coverage in the new outpatient prescription drug plan, there is not the usual "stop-loss" provision (limiting a person's financial liability) that is associated with most other insurance coverage. As a result, almost 90 percent of seniors have coverage in addition to Medicare, obtained from various sources such as employers, supplementary Medigap, Medicare Advantage, or Medicaid.[1] This supplementary coverage generally shields seniors from the deductibles associated with Parts A and B, as well as the 20 percent coinsurance associated with Part B expenditures. Nonetheless, even with Medicare and supplementary insurance, almost 20 percent of seniors' health care is financed out of pocket.[2]

The difference between the benefit packages for the Medicare population and the under-65 population primarily reflects differences in the expected use of benefits, particularly with the addition of outpatient prescription drug coverage to Medicare benefits. The difference in the financial orientation of the delivery system for each group reflects differences in financial incentives and funding liabilities between the two populations.

In the under-65 population, for whom most insurance is sponsored by employers, premiums are paid by employers and employees. Costs for managed care or network plans are usually less than those for indemnity plans. The more loosely organized networks, like Point of Service (POS) or Preferred Provider Organizations (PPOs), are more expensive than health maintenance organizations (HMOs), and network plans of all sorts cost less than old-fashioned indemnity plans, which have pretty much disappeared for the under-65 population.[3] Hence, most of the under-65 population is enrolled in some type of managed care or network plan. In contrast, most seniors are in the traditional fee-for-service indemnity program.

Private plan participation in Medicare has varied substantially during the last fifteen years but has never represented a very large portion of the senior population. Private plan participation reached a maximum of 17 percent of the Medicare population, but following the passage of the Balanced Budget Act of 1997, many plans withdrew from at least some areas of the country, and participation dropped to 12 percent by the end of 2003.[4] Following passage of the Medicare Modernization Act (MMA) in 2003, enrollment has started growing again. By December 2005, 14 percent of beneficiaries were enrolled in private plans.[5]

Private plan options increased in 2006, in part as a result of the requirement that seniors enroll in a private plan to receive the new drug benefit (although not necessarily to receive other Medicare benefits). It is too soon to know whether the growth experienced in 2005 will continue or whether private plans will show as much interest in participating in Medicare as they have in the past few years. If the capitation rate is reduced, perhaps to find funds for other purposes, future growth may be less robust.

Similar to spending throughout the health care sector, spending in the Medicare program is highly concentrated. In 2002, 5 percent of the program's population accounted for almost half of fee-for-service spending, and 25 percent of the population accounted for almost 90 percent of spending.[6] Medicare spending is actually slightly less concentrated than spending for the under-65 population because the level of spending for all seniors is so much higher than that of the under-65 population. Over one-quarter of Medicare spending occurs during the last year of a beneficiary's life, a number that has held constant for several decades. Medicare beneficiaries use a disproportionate amount of health care relative to their numbers, reflecting both the greater prevalence of chronic conditions and the higher mortality among the elderly.[7]

Medicare versus the Rest of Health Care

In Medicare, the incentives to moderate spending or change behavior have been placed predominantly on the providers. Although beneficiaries spend substantial amounts of money out of pocket on health care, primarily for services not covered by Medicare, they tend to face small or no price increases for Medicare-covered services between what Medicare pays and what their supplementary insurance pays. With minimal pricing concerns at the point of use, most beneficiaries face few constraints in their use of, or access to, health services—except those who live in areas with limited health care capacity or where physicians are refusing Medicare patients.

Medicare's provider incentives vary according to the service covered. For hospital stays and nursing home and home care services, payments are made for a bundle of services under Medicare's prospective pricing systems. Under bundled payments, the incentive is to provide fewer and less costly services within the services covered by the payment—by being more efficient, by skimping on services, or by selecting patients healthier than the average. There is also an incentive to increase the number of bundled payments by readmitting patients to hospitals or providing multiple episodes of home care. In addition, although the reimbursement is nominally based on the diagnosis, it is also affected by the treatment. Thus bypass surgery is reimbursed differently than angioplasty, although both may be reflecting a similar disease state.

For services priced according to a fee schedule under Medicare, such as the relative value scale used for physician services, providers have an incentive to increase the volume of services, especially for those that are highly compensated relative to their costs. Even though the sustainable growth rate ties total physician spending under Medicare to growth in the economy, thus providing an overall restraint on physician spending, the incentive for any individual physician remains to increase volume.

Medicare does not reward quality care or improved clinical outcomes. This is true for institutional providers who receive bundled payments and individual clinicians who are paid according to a fee schedule.

The incentives in the private sector are more diverse because of substantial variation in reimbursement and insurance used, although many insurance companies use Medicare-like reimbursement strategies for providers. Unlike Medicare, pressure to moderate spending is distributed more broadly in the private sector. Enrollees covered by private insurance frequently have a co-payment or coinsurance for at least some services; they may face different financial incentives toward in-network and out-of-network use; and a relatively small number are now enrolled in high-deductible plans that are often paired with a tax-favored medical savings account.

Providers also face a variety of incentives. Many plans use bundled payment systems, resembling those in Medicare, particularly for hospital payments. Some plans also use multiples of Medicare's relative value scale, while other plans use their own fee schedules. As in Medicare, there are frequently implicit incentives to increase the volume of services provided, few incentives for efficiency other than those associated with a bundled payment, and no rewards for quality care or clinical outcomes.

Innovative Strategies

Both private payers and Medicare understand the importance of changing some of the perverse incentives facing providers. There are more than 100 different pay-for-performance (P4P) experiments underway in the private sector and two large Medicare demonstrations in progress—with several others just beginning—that attempt to reward quality and encourage efficiency.[8]

The hospital pilot project of Premier Inc. focuses on rewarding quality. Hospitals in the top 10 percent on quality measures receive a 2 percent increase to their diagnosis-related group (DRG) reimbursement; those in the next 10 percent receive a 1 percent increase. In the third year of the demonstration, penalties are being imposed on any hospital that has not exceeded the bottom 20 percent in quality from the baseline of the pilot's first year. Early reports indicate that participating hospitals had larger increases in quality improvement than did nonparticipating hospitals. Equally promising are reports indicating lower costs for at least some medical conditions.[9]

Medicare is also sponsoring a group practice demonstration that focuses on quality and efficiency by allowing practices whose patients show at least 2 percentage points slower growth in expenditures—compared with what other beneficiaries in their area spend—to keep 80 percent of the savings above the 2 percent threshold. This demonstration is still in its early stages, and thus relatively limited results are available.[10]

The Medicare Health Support pilot program, a care management demonstration, could help moderate spending for high-cost beneficiaries with complex needs. It is a chronic care improvement program for patients in fee-for-service Medicare with congestive heart failure or diabetes. Organizations providing care for these patients are paid a fee by the Centers for Medicare and Medicaid Services (CMS) for care coordination. Retaining the fee is contingent on demonstrating prespecified levels of savings.[11]

An additional demonstration scheduled to begin in 2007 allows for "gainsharing" between physicians and hospitals that are not part of integrated delivery systems. Various methodologies will be tested that allow hospitals to share savings with the physicians who produce them, thus providing for a better alignment of incentives between hospitals and physicians than exists under traditional Medicare. As in the other demonstrations, participants will be required to maintain or improve quality while demonstrating cost savings. Unlike current law, hospitals will be able to share up to 25 percent of the documented cost savings from quality improvements with physicians.[12]

These demonstrations may provide successfully tested strategies to improve performance that can be introduced into the full Medicare program. The inclusion of small and medium-sized physician practices, as well as demonstrations that focus on fee-for-service, is especially important because it is representative of most physicians' practices and how most beneficiaries receive care. Unfortunately, in the past many successful demonstrations have proved difficult to implement at the national level, although the results of some demonstrations have affected changes in Medicare reimbursement structures. Because of the extraordinary importance of saving resources and improving quality in the Medicare program, it is possible that the experience of these demonstrations will be different. At the very least, they will provide important information about whether these types of changes would be desirable, information which would be available if and when the political will is found to introduce such changes.

Medicare versus the Private Sector: Who Has Been More Successful Moderating Spending?

There is ongoing debate about whether Medicare or the private sector has been more successful in restraining health care spending. When considering relatively small, discrete blocks of time, rates of growth in per capita spending can indeed differ between Medicare and private insurance. For example, from the early 1990s until the 1997 passage of the Balanced Budget Act, private insurance grew slower than Medicare. Since 1997, Medicare has been growing slower—sometimes substantially—than private insurance.

Some researchers claim that Medicare has been more successful over the last twenty years, beginning with the phase-in of bundled payments for hospitals.[13] The Medicare Payment Advisory Commission (MedPAC) reports that during the period from 1970 to 2002, Medicare spending has grown about 1 percentage point slower than private insurance (excluding outpatient prescription drugs so that the benefits are more comparable). However, during that same period private-sector benefits expanded and cost-sharing requirements declined, while Medicare benefits remained relatively unchanged.[14] Although it is difficult to make adequate adjustments to judge spending streams on a comparable benefits basis, an appropriate comparison of the spending streams cannot be made without such adjustments.[15]

Politically, the notion that Medicare could sustain lower rates of spending growth for any extended period relative to private insurance— implying less access to new technology, less or differential access to high-priced providers, or differential efficiencies by providers—seems totally untenable. Medicare is currently the country's single largest payer of health care services. The impending retirement of the baby boomers will double the Medicare beneficiary population under current law. When baby boomer retirement is coupled with the increasing population share that those over 65 will represent, the likelihood that the Medicare growth rate can deviate from that of private insurance is even less tenable in the future than it is now. It is highly unlikely that middle-class seniors would tolerate sustained differences that produced what they perceived as inferior or undesirable results, assuming they continue not having to pay the full cost of the services.

This does not mean that Medicare or the private sector cannot each lead at different times regarding change. That can and does happen, but spending streams tend to converge over time. Thus sustaining a lower rate of spending growth per capita in Medicare will only happen if there is a comparable rate of spending growth in the private sector.

Objectives of Reform

The objectives for a reformed Medicare program may vary depending on one's political values and views on political feasibility. Here, four objectives are suggested to guide transformation of the program:

—Protect the most vulnerable among the aged and disabled.

—Begin reform as soon as politically possible to allow for as much transition time as possible.

—Move to substantially moderate the growth in spending.

—Find ways to improve the value of health care provided and received.

Menu of Options

Numerous analysts from across the political spectrum have estimated the budget effects of different strategies to slow Medicare spending. Some of these changes are attractive on policy grounds as well as for their budgetary effect, others primarily for their budgetary effects.

In reviewing the various options, this section follows the taxonomy used by MedPAC in their 2006 report, which includes the following:

—constraining payments

—limiting benefits and changing cost sharing, including increasing the age of eligibility

—increasing program financing

—increasing efficiency, including improving incentives within fee-for-service, using private plans to deliver Medicare benefits, and competing with traditional Medicare

—realigning incentives within Medicare, more broadly within health care including differential payments to providers, improved incentives for patients, and the development of comparative effectiveness information

Constraining payments is the most frequently used strategy to slow down Medicare spending. Each year, Congress decides whether and how much to update the various payments to providers. The Balanced Budget Act of 1997 aggressively slowed payments to providers for a short time, but as experience has shown, it is very difficult to sustain these slowdowns over time, especially if the drivers of spending are not addressed and spending in the private sector does not follow suit. After two years of unexpectedly slow spending growth, Congress "gave back" some of the savings, and Medicare spending is now projected to grow at a rate of 7.3 percent per year over the next decade.

It may be impossible to lower spending by constraining payments if volume or intensity of services or both are increasing. The importance of volume can be seen in Part B spending where, in 2005, physician fees increased at a rate of only 1.5 percent while Part B spending increased by 15 percent. The Congressional Budget Office (CBO) has estimated five-year savings for a variety of payment constraints (see appendix). Although they are modestly helpful in reducing Medicare expenditures in the short term, they have little appreciable effect on the problem. In addition, while some have argued that prices are a big part of the problem in the United States, reducing prices would represent more of a one-off saving than it would a reduction in the growth rate in spending, which is the larger challenge.[16] In addition, unless medical prices are reduced everywhere, it would be difficult to sustain the difference over time.

Limiting benefits—by increasing Medicare's age of eligibility, expanding beneficiary cost sharing, or limiting the benefit coverage—is not likely to be politically popular, at least not among the Medicare beneficiary population, but it could have more sustained financial impact.

Increasing the eligibility age to 67 to make Medicare eligibility consistent with Social Security has been raised as a strategy for improving Medicare's financial position. Part of the appeal of this approach lies in the continuing increase in longevity being experienced by the American population. Current life expectancy in this country is 77.6 years. In 2003 American men could expect to live three years longer, and women more than one year longer, than they did in 1990.[17]

Increasing the eligibility age would reduce Medicare spending. However, the reduction may be less than presumed since the youngest beneficiaries tend to have lower than average medical expenditures.[18] The amount of savings will also depend on how quickly the age of eligibility is increased. If implementation follows Social Security and increases age eligibility by 2 months a year beginning in 2015, it would reduce spending only by 0.2 percent by 2075. If the eligibility age continued to increase by two months per year to age 70, the savings would be 0.8 percent of GDP by 2078.[19] A more rapid rise in eligibility age could occur if substantial advance warning were provided.

Increasing beneficiary cost sharing could provide significant revenues in the short term—CBO estimates that increasing the beneficiaries share of Part B from 25 to 35 percent would reduce spending by approximately $85 billion over the next decade.[20] However, concern has been raised that an across-the-board increase could impose financial hardships on lower-income beneficiaries and could also discourage the use of some medically necessary services.[21]

In addition, the Medicare Modernization Act will already substantially reduce the Part B subsidy for higher-income beneficiaries starting in 2007, with changes phased in over three years. Individuals with annual incomes of at least $80,000 will pay an income-based surcharge on the monthly premium. There is discussion on whether or not additional cost sharing would begin to result in fewer enrollees, but under current rules, Medicare continues to offer a substantial subsidy even for the highest-income individuals, and estimates of seniors dropping out of the program tend to be very small. For example, of the 1.8 million individuals who will be affected by the phased-in changes that start in 2007, it has been estimated that only 30,000 will drop out of the program.[22] Thus, relating income to other parts of Medicare is likely to be raised in the future as Medicare expenditures place increasingly greater pressure on the Part A trust fund and on the general revenues used to finance Parts B and D.

MedPAC and others have suggested combining increased cost sharing with stop-loss or catastrophic coverage. This is an old idea, variants of which date back to proposals in the Reagan administration. It makes policy sense but gives back some of the savings. If combined with a prohibition on supplementary insurance, however, it could both alter behavior and save money. Banning supplementary insurance for Medicare to maintain financial incentives associated with cost sharing is a perennial favorite among economists and policy analysts but lacks political saliency in the extreme.

Limiting Medicare's coverage could also reduce spending, but this would have appeal only if done selectively or if combined with information on clinical effectiveness. "Tiering" coinsurance according to the appropriateness of use is a more attractive potential strategy. Limiting Medicare's coverage more generally and across the board is not very attractive given the substantial share of health care spending already not covered by Medicare.

Given the increasing share of GDP that will be going to Medicare, even if Medicare spending is able to grow at a level closer to 1 percent above GDP, enhancing program funding is likely to be a part of any long-term strategy to reform and bring into balance Medicare's funding and spending projections. However, increasing program funding alone does not address the imperative to slow Medicare spending as part of an overall strategy to restore fiscal sanity.

One option that may hold more promise is to moderate spending by increasing efficiency. While traditionally MedPAC has focused on whether the payments made to Medicare providers represent adequate reimbursement for efficient providers, MedPAC, CMS, and other payers and analysts increasingly have recognized that payments to providers under Medicare offer, at most, only limited incentives to achieving efficiency and no reward for producing quality or appropriate clinical outcomes.

As important as it is to change reimbursement systems to drive changes in provider behavior, it would also be helpful if beneficiaries were rewarded or presented with incentives to use health care more efficiently. This latter objective underlies the movement towards consumer-directed health plans. It focuses not only on giving financial incentives to patients to be more cost conscious while using care but also on driving greater transparency in pricing and quality information. Another way to encourage seniors to be more cost conscious is to change the incentives they face when choosing their health plan. One of the frequently cited ways to do this is to adopt the model of the Federal Employees Health Benefits program of plan selection in which the government contribution does not vary with the cost of the plan. In Medicare, this strategy has also been called the premium support model.[23]

The increased use of bundled payments in reimbursing Medicare services—rather than paying for specific inputs of care—represented an important change that was first introduced by Medicare in the 1980s. It has been increasingly adopted by private-sector payers. Bundled payments are currently used for inpatient and outpatient hospital reimbursement, for home care, and to a lesser degree for nursing homes. Under bundled payments, institutions can capture the results of being efficient if they can provide care at less than the average cost represented by the bundled payment. However, there has been ongoing concern regarding potential gaming through "upcoding," that is, increasing the code to increase the complexity and therefore the payment.

The incentive for efficiency associated with bundled payments does not exist for physicians under Medicare. The use of a relative value–based fee schedule that ties updates to the aggregate level of spending on Part B provides no opportunity for efficient physicians to gain rewards.

However, neither the bundled payment method of reimbursement nor the disaggregated physician fee schedule provides any reward for quality or improved clinical outcomes. The lack of a reward for quality, the limited rewards for efficiency, and the recognition that there are very wide variations in spending levels that appear either to not be associated with different outcomes or to have a perverse association have led to calls for a fundamental revamping of reimbursement to providers under Medicare.

The systemically unhelpful incentives in Medicare reimbursements are generally present in the private sector and are driving much of the interest in implementing some type of pay-for-performance (P4P) reimbursement system there as well. As discussed earlier, both CMS and the private sector are in the process of experimenting with different strategies that reward quality and improved outcomes, either independent of savings or as a result of the savings.

Pay-for-performance strategies attempt to realign incentives both to encourage ongoing improvement in the delivery of health care and to reward those who produce efficient, high quality care. These strategies pay for results instead of paying for the volume and intensity of specific services, regardless of the outcomes they produce or the appropriateness of the care delivered. However, many changes need to occur and many questions need to be addressed before a pay-for-performance system could be introduced into Medicare.

The first requirement is the development of a national performance measurement system that could be used as a basis for redesigning a payment system. The Institute of Medicine (IOM) has recently released a report entitled *Performance Measurement: Accelerating Improvement* that assesses the current state of performance measurement and recommends strategies to develop a usable performance measurement system for the future.[24]

The many decisions that need to be made to enable full implementation of P4P include how to reward improvement and attainment in some weighted manner, how to phase in a pay-for-performance system, how much of the reimbursement should or must reflect pay-for-performance to have an impact on behavior, whether to use new or existing Medicare funds, and how to adjust for differences in health status and compliance. The latter is particularly important to minimize the incentive to choose healthier patients or to further disadvantage safety net facilities that may have unusually high numbers of sicker or less compliant patients.

Moving to a payment system that encourages and rewards efficiency and quality improvement is an important part of any "spending smarter" strategy. However, it will take time to put in place because there is so much currently unknown and untested. During the phase-in of a new reimbursement system, it will be important to conduct ongoing assessment of the effects of changes to the reimbursement system. Recognizing the amount of change that needs to occur, IOM has recommended engaging in what it has termed "active learning," that is, adjusting and undertaking corrective actions in response to undesired or unintended consequences.[25]

Realigning incentives so that providers are encouraged to work collaboratively to improve the quality and efficiency of health care, and are
rewarded for doing so, is the first component to "spending smarter." A
second component is to develop good comparative clinical information
on the effectiveness of medical procedures and technologies, so that
providers, payers, and consumers can better understand the likely effects
of using a particular therapeutic device or medical technology for a
patient with a given set of symptoms and risk factors. To date, most of the
interest in comparative effectiveness information has been directed
toward pharmaceuticals and occasionally new devices. Although these
are important areas of health care with many innovative and often expensive products that require coverage and reimbursement decisions, the
potential payoff for better decision-making is even greater in other areas
of health care, particularly the broader area of medical procedures.[26]

Determining the appropriate function, placement, structure, and
financing of a comparative effectiveness center in the United States raises
significant questions about the appropriate role of government. In most
countries, information on comparative effectiveness and cost effectiveness has been used to make coverage and reimbursement decisions as part
of the national health plan. In the United States, the more appropriate
function of a comparative effectiveness center would be to provide credible, objective information that any payer could use. The expectation is
that different payers would use the information differently, in terms of
structuring differential reimbursement or co-payment rates based on comparative clinical effectiveness, but that the availability of the information
is critical for payers, providers, and patients to make better decisions.[27]

What would happen if the United States invested in making credible
clinical information available on comparative effectiveness for at least
the highest-cost, highest-volume procedures and technologies—an
investment that would likely require expenditures of at least $4 billion to
$6 billion on an annualized basis for many years—and if it adopted a
payment-for-results model of reimbursement that aligned incentives
across various providers to encourage the delivery of coordinated, effective, and efficient health care? Such action would certainly improve the
value of care received, but it is unclear whether spending growth rates
would be modified. There would be many "one-off" savings that could

reduce the absolute level of spending per person and increase the value of health care spending. It seems reasonable that a realignment of incentives coupled with better information will also moderate spending growth rates, but it is not possible to know for certain whether and how much change in growth rates would result unless and until this approach is tried. However, given the other options available, which would either have little impact or seem politically infeasible, moving in the direction of providing credible clinical information and rewarding results seems very compelling.

Where Can Medicare and the Federal Government Lead and Where Must Medicare Follow?

The federal government can and should take the lead investing in the development and public availability of comparative effectiveness information. This type of information can be regarded as a traditional public good in the way economists use that term—once available, its use does not diminish its availability to other users; it is not excludable. This is clearly an important area for government leadership, regardless of whether or not there could be some joint financing with the private sector or placement in a quasi-government center to encourage the trust and buy-in of the private sector. Because the Medicare program will clearly be an important beneficiary of such information, Medicare could reasonably be regarded as a financial contributor to this activity, so long as the financing does not come exclusively out of general revenues.

It is more complicated to determine whether the government and Medicare can take the lead in realigning reimbursement to reward those who provide efficient, high quality care—that is, paying for results instead of paying for what is nominally the same service. Historically, Medicare has had great difficulty introducing concepts of selective contracting or competitive bidding in health care—both concepts that the private sector has used liberally since the 1980s. Even in areas with minimal service components, like durable medical equipment, competitive bidding has been difficult to introduce. Although it was first considered in 1992, competitive bidding for durable equipment is only now being phased in, from 2007 to 2009.

At the very least, Medicare can sponsor extensive experimentation involving different models of pay-for-performance, as it is now doing with the various current, or soon to be operating, demonstrations. These demonstrations include assessments of the sensitivity of various types of providers to differential payment strategies, the unintended consequences associated with different payment strategies, and implementation issues. Medicare could also help disseminate the knowledge produced by the demonstrations. CMS can and should also continue to be part of consortiums like NCQA (the National Committee for Quality Assurance) and NQF (the National Quality Forum).

It is possible that if the formulas used to calculate the pay-for-performance strategies appear "rigorous enough," or are at least objectively defined so that they appear more like diagnosis-related groups (DRGs) and the Resource-Based Relative Value Scale (RBRVS), Medicare may be able to take the lead in introducing payment realignment. Particularly in the current atmosphere, where there is significant interest in bailing out physicians from anticipated fee reductions over the next several years, it may be possible to phase in a pay-for-performance strategy that would begin with pay for reporting, as was done for hospitals following the Medicare Modernization Act. Other sectors in Medicare, such as hospitals, renal dialysis centers, and Medicare Advantage plans, are close to being ready to begin a phase-in of pay-for-performance, if the political will exists to move in this direction.

Even if the political will does exist, there are advantages and disadvantages to having Medicare take the lead. The advantage is that a large part of the health care sector would move toward paying for outcomes and results. The primary concern, however, is that the introduction of such a system and any subsequent changes will require new statutory language that would have to be implemented through the regulatory process. This whole area is very much in flux, and using the statutory and regulatory mechanisms of the federal government is a cumbersome, inflexible process.

Thus it is important to at least raise the question of whether it is too early in the evolution of a realigned reimbursement system for the government to take the lead in introducing it, even if it is politically possible to do so. The trade-off is balancing the use of government's power and ability to make things happen quickly and in a significant way versus the ability of the private sector to be nimble, flexible, and "quicker on its feet." On balance, if Medicare can begin introducing pay-for-performance components into its reimbursement system, it should do so in a careful and phased process. The private sector should continue to follow suit, as it is doing sporadically now, and should pursue some of the innovations that appear necessary after early findings from the Medicare program.

Sensible Next Steps

Finding ways to slow the growth rate in Medicare spending, and thus in the rest of health care—given the historical ways in which they have trended together and the likelihood that this trending will become even more important in the future—is even more urgent following the introduction of the Part D drug benefit than it has been in the past.

Sensible next steps include the following:

—Move as quickly as politically and technically possible toward changing and realigning financial incentives for providers and, to the extent feasible, making patients more conscious of cost and quality.

—Improve the availability of comparative information on effectiveness.

—Introduce more competitive elements into Medicare.

—Provide full benefits for those with health-related disabilities and begin to gradually increase the age for full benefits for those without health-related disabilities.

—Extend the Medicare principle of relating incomes to premiums beyond Part B. How and how much will depend on whether the dominance of the fee-for-service system continues in the future and on how far relating incomes to premiums can go before people at the high end of the income scale start to rebel or push back.

Although there are no guarantees that these steps would actually reduce growth rates in spending, they represent a combination of reasonable next steps that could imaginably survive the test of political feasibility. Making more and better information available and realigning financial incentives seem to be among the few areas that have garnered both bipartisan and bicameral interest. That does not, however, mean their passage would be easy. As any former or current administrator of the Health Care Financing Administration or the Centers for Medicare and Medicaid Services can attest, nothing big in Medicare happens easily.

Appendix[a]

Budget options— Constraining payments	Potential savings	Details of option
Remove Medicare's payments for indirect medical education (IME) from the benchmarks for private plans.	$326 million in 2006 and $2.1 billion over 5 years	Remove payments for IME from the benchmarks for private plans, leaving the payment to teaching hospitals as the only compensation for IME.
Reduce Medicare's direct payments for graduate medical education (GME).	2004 costs totaled $2.2 billion; savings are $800 million in 2006 and $4.6 billion over 5 years	GME direct payments would be set at 120 percent of the national average salary paid to residents in 1987, updated annually for changes in consumer prices; option would reduce teaching and overhead payments while continuing to pay residents' compensation; would pay each hospital the same amount for the same type of resident.
Reduce Medicare's payments for the indirect costs of patient care related to hospitals' teaching programs.	$2.9 billion in 2006 and $17.2 billion over 5 years	Lower the IME adjustment to 2.7 percent from 5.5 percent for every increase of 0.1 in the ratio of full-time residents to number of beds.
Equalize Medicare's capital-related payments for teaching and nonteaching hospitals.	$400 million in 2006 and $2.4 billion over 5 years	Eliminate extra payments to teaching hospitals.
Convert Medicare's payments for GME into a block grant and slow their growth.	$600 million in 2006 and $3.3 billion over 5 years	Replaces current payment system with consolidated block grant to fund all GME activities at teaching hospitals (see three options above).

Budget options— Constraining payments	Potential savings	Details of option
Convert Medicare's dispro-portionate share of hospi-tal (DSH) payments into a block grant.	$1.2 billion in 2006 and $10.5 billion over 5 years	Converts DSH payments into a block grant to the states. In 2006 each grant would be 10 percent less than the estimated sum of Medicare DSH payments made to hospitals in that state in 2005. In subsequent years, the grant would be indexed to the change in the con-sumer price index (CPI) for all urban consumers minus 1 percentage point. States would be given flexibility in how they used their DSH funds.
Reduce the update factor for hospital inpatient operating costs under Medicare.	$1.2 billion in 2008 and $55 billion through 2015 (over 10 years)	Reduces the Medicare prospective payment sys-tem (PPS) update factor to the annual change in the Medicaid Buy-In (MBI) minus 1 percentage point. Rate would take effect in 2008 and continue through at least 2015.
Reduce Medicare's pay-ments for hospital inpa-tient capital-related costs.	$400 million in 2006 and $2.4 billion over 5 years	Would further reduce the prospective payment rate for hospitals' capital-related costs by 5 percent-age points—bringing the total reduction to about 22 percent from the initial level.
Reduce Medicare's pay-ments for home health care.	$240 million in 2006 and $6.3 billion over 5 years	Freeze the base payment for each home health episode at its calendar year 2005 level ($2,264) through 2009, with the goal of gradually narrowing the gap between payments and costs.

Budget options— Constraining payments	Potential savings	Details of option
Raise the eligibility age for Medicare.	0.2 percent to 0.8 percent of GDP by 2075	Two alternatives: increase eligibility age by 2 months every year beginning in 2015 until it reached 67 in 2026; increase eligibility age same as above but until it reached 70 in 2044.
Increase Medicare's premium for supplementary medical insurance (SMI) to 30 percent of benefit costs.	$4.7 billion in 2006 and $33.5 billion over 5 years	Set the SMI premium equal to 30 percent of the cost of Part B benefits; would raise the 2006 premium for enrollees to $95.70 per month versus $79.80.
Restructure Medicare's cost-sharing requirements.	$4.7 billion in 2006 and $34.3 billion over 5 years	Replace the current complicated mix of cost-sharing provisions with a single combined deductible covering all services in Parts A and B of Medicare, a uniform coinsurance rate of 20 percent for amounts above that deductible (including inpatient expenses), and an annual cap on each beneficiary's total cost-sharing liabilities. Combined deductible would be $500 in 2006, and the cap on total cost sharing would be $4,500 in later years. Those amounts would grow at the same rate as per capita Medicare costs.
Restrict Medigap coverage of Medicare's cost sharing.	$2.1 billion in 2006 and $15.8 billion over 5 years	Bar Medigap policies from paying any of the first $500 of an enrollee's cost-sharing liabilities for calendar year 2006 and limit coverage to 50 percent of the next $4,000 in Medicare cost sharing.

Budget options— Constraining payments	Potential savings	Details of option
Combine changes to Medicare's cost sharing with Medigap restrictions.	$7.1 billion in 2006 and $52.2 billion over 5 years	Medigap plans would be prohibited from covering any of the new $500 combined deductible that would be required by Medicare in 2006 and could cover only 50 percent of the program's remaining cost-sharing requirements.
Impose a co-payment requirement on home health episodes covered by Medicare.	$1.5 billion in 2006 and $11.8 billion over 5 years	Charge beneficiaries a co-payment amounting to 10 percent of the total cost of each home health "episode"—a 60-day period of services—covered by Medicare, starting on January 1, 2006.
Impose cost sharing for the first 20 days of a skilled nursing facility stay under Medicare.	$1.1 billion in 2006 and $8 billion over 5 years	Impose a co-payment for the first 20 days of care in a skilled nursing facility equal to 5 percent of the inpatient deductible, which would be $47.20 per day in 2006. Maximum additional liability for a beneficiary would thus equal the inpatient deductible and would rise at the same rate over time.
Impose a deductible and coinsurance amounts for clinical laboratory services under Medicare.	$800 million in 2006 and $5.9 billion over 5 years	Impose the SMI program's usual deductible and coinsurance requirements on laboratory services, beginning Jan 1, 2006.

a. Cost estimates based on Congressional Budget Office, "570: Medicare," in *Budget Options* (GPO: February 2005), pp. 191–215 (www.cbo.gov/showdoc.cfm?index=6075&sequence=13). Because of interactions among policies, the net savings that could be gained by adopting a combination of options is likely to be lower than the sum of the parts.

Notes

1. Kaiser Family Foundation and Health Research and Educational Trust, *Medicare Chartbook*, 3d ed. (Menlo, Calif.: Henry J. Kaiser Family Foundation and Chicago: HRET, summer 2005) (www.kff.org/medicare/7284.cfm).

2. Kaiser Family Foundation, *Medicare Chartbook*, p. 33, figure 4-1 "Sources of Payment for Medicare Beneficiaries' Medical and Long Term Care Services, 2002." Medicare pays 45 percent, Medicaid 12 percent, private insurance 18 percent, direct out-of-pocket 19 percent, and other sources 6 percent.

3. Kaiser Family Foundation and Health Research and Educational Trust, *Employer Health Benefits: 2005 Annual Survey,* "Summary of Findings" (2005) (www.kff.org/insurance/7315/upload/7315.pdf).

4. Douglas Holtz-Eakin, CBO director, "Health Care Spending and the Uninsured," statement before the Committee on Health, Education, Labor, and Pensions, U.S. Senate, 108th Cong., 2nd sess. (Washington, January 28, 2004) (www.cbo.gov/ftpdocs/49xx/doc4989/01-28-HealthTestimony.pdf).

5. Stephanie Peterson and Marsha Gold, "Tracking Medicare Health and Prescription Drug Plans: Monthly Report for January 2006," Report 82 (Mathematica Policy Research for Kaiser Family Foundation, February 1, 2006) (http://www.kff.org/medicare/upload/medicaretracking0106.pdf).

6. MedPAC, *Report to the Congress: New Approaches in Medicare* (Washington: Medicare Payment Advisory Commission, June 2004).

7. MedPAC, *Report to the Congress: Medicare Payment Policy* (March 2005); Gerard F. Anderson, Biana K. Frogner, Roger A. Johns, and Uwe E. Reinhardt, "Health Care Spending and Use of Information Technology in OECD Countries," *Health Affairs* 25, no. 3 (May-June 2006): 819–31.

8. Institute of Medicine (IOM), Board on Health Care Services, *Performance Measurement: Accelerating Improvement* (Washington: National Academies Press, 2006); Centers for Medicare & Medicaid Services, "Medicare Begins Performance-Based Payments for Physician Groups," press release, January 31, 2005 (www.cms.hhs.gov/apps/media/press/release.asp?Counter=1341); CMS, "Medicare Demonstration Shows Hospital Quality of Care Improves with Payments Tied to Quality," press release, November 14, 2005 (www.cms.hhs.gov/apps/media/press/release.asp?Counter=1729).

9. Stephanie Alexander, "CMS/Premier Hospital Quality Incentive Demonstration Project: 1st Year Results," paper prepared for the IOM P4P subcommittee meeting, Washington, November 30, 2005 (Charlotte, N.C.: Premier, Inc.).

10. CMS, "Medicare Health Support: Overview" (July 2006) (www.cms.hhs.gov/CCIP/01_Overview.asp#TopOfPage).

11. Ibid.

12. CMS, Medicare Demonstrations, "Physician-Hospital Collaboration Demonstration," September 7, 2006 (www.cms.hhs.gov/DemoProjectsEval Rpts/MD/itemdetail.asp?filterType=none&filterByDID=-99&sortbyDID=3&sort Order=ascending&itemID=CMS1186653).

13. Cristina Boccuti and Marilyn Moon, "Comparing Medicare and Private Insurers: Growth Rates in Spending Over Three Decades," *Health Affairs* 22, no. 2 (March-April 2003): 230–37.

14. MedPAC, *A Data Book: Healthcare Spending and the Medicare Program*, section 1: "National Health Care and Medicare Spending" (June 2006) (www. medpac.gov/publications/congressional_reports/Jun06DataBookSec1.pdf).

15. Joseph R. Antos, "The Role of Market Competition in Strengthening Medicare," testimony before the Senate Special Committee on Aging, 108th Cong., 1st sess. (Washington: American Enterprise Institute, May 6, 2003).

16. Gerard F. Anderson, Uwe E. Reinhardt, Peter S. Hussey, and Varduhi Petrosyan, "It's The Prices, Stupid: Why the United States Is So Different from Other Countries," *Health Affairs* 22, no. 3 (May-June 2003): 89–105.

17. National Center for Health Statistics, Centers for Disease Control and Prevention, *Health, United States, 2005 with Chartbook on Trends in the Health of Americans* (Washington: Government Printing Office, 2005) (www.cdc.gov/nchs/data/hus/hus05.pdf#027); Congressional Budget Office, *Budget Options* (Washington, February 2005) (www.cbo.gov/showdoc.cfm?index=6075&sequence=0& from=0#anchor).

18. The greater impact of raising the eligibility age is to encourage greater labor force participation, which could reduce dependence on entitlements and add to revenue.

19. CBO, *Budget Options*.

20. MedPAC, *Report to the Congress: Medicare Payment Policy* (March 2006) (www.medpac.gov/publications/congressional_reports/Mar06_TOC.pdf).

21. Ibid.; Thomas Rice and Karen Y. Matsuoka, "The Impact of Cost Sharing on Appropriate Utilization and Health Status: A Review of the Literature on Seniors," *Medical Care Research and Review* 61, no. 4 (December 2004): 415–52.

22. Kaiser Family Foundation, Daily Health Policy Report, "Medicare: Medicare Part B Premiums to Rise 5.6 Percent Next Year; Seniors with Higher Incomes to Pay More" (September 13, 2006) (www.kaisernetwork.org/daily_reports/rep_index.cfm?hint=3&DR_ID=39770).

23. Henry Aaron and Robert Reischauer, "The Medicare Reform Debate: What Is the Next Step?" *Health Affairs* 14, no. 4 (Winter 1995): 8–30; Gail R. Wilensky and Joseph P. Newhouse, "Medicare: What's Right? What's Wrong? What's Next?" *Health Affairs* 18, no. 1 (January-February 1999): 92–106.

24. IOM, *Performance Measurement: Accelerating Improvement*.

25. IOM, Committee on Redesigning Health Insurance Performance Measures, Payment, and Performance Improvement Programs, *Rewarding Provider Performance: Aligning Incentives in Medicare* (Washington: National Academies Press, 2006)

26. Gail R. Wilensky, "Developing a Center for Comparative Effectiveness Information," *Health Affairs* web exclusive, November 7, 2006: W572–W585 (summary: www.cmwf.org/usr_doc/Wilensky_develctrcompareffect_967_itl.pdf).

27. Ibid.

4

The Role of Medicaid

ALAN R. WEIL AND LOUIS F. ROSSITER

Any serious efforts to control the federal budget must include Medicaid. Although the share of the federal budget devoted to Medicaid is substantially smaller than that for Medicare, the anticipated rate of growth in Medicaid is slightly higher than that for Medicare and substantially above anticipated growth in federal revenues. Medicaid dominates the markets for some services and can help move the health system toward greater efficiency by serving as a model for effective delivery.

Medicaid spending is expected to grow for the same reasons health care spending is expected to grow—advances in medical technology and increasing needs of the population—but Medicaid is also affected by forces unique to it. Those forces are the focus of this chapter.

Medicaid's Place in Budgets and the Health System

While the federal government struggles with Medicaid spending, the states struggle even more. The federal government spent $181.5 billion on Medicaid in 2005, while the states spent $133.6 billion (table 4-1).

Table 4-1. *National Health Expenditures (NHE), by Source of Funds, Amounts, and Average Annual Growth from Prior Year Shown, Selected Calendar Years 1993–2015*[a]

Source of funds (billions of dollars)	1993	2002	2003	2004	2005[b]	2006[b]	2010[b]	2015[b]
NHE	916.5	1,607.9	1,740.6	1,877.6	2,016.0	2,163.9	2,879.4	4,031.7
Private funds	514.2	881.4	957.2	1,030.3	1,101.4	1,148.4	1,544.7	2,116.4
Consumer payments	442.3	763.0	829.7	894.2	955.2	991.2	1,334.1	1,818.1
Out-of-pocket payments	145.3	210.8	223.5	235.7	248.8	246.2	316.3	421.0
Private health insurance	297.0	552.2	606.3	658.5	706.4	745.0	1,017.7	1,397.1
Other private funds	71.9	118.4	127.5	136.1	146.2	157.1	210.6	298.3
Public funds	402.3	726.5	783.4	847.3	914.6	1,015.5	1,334.7	1,915.3
Federal	277.7	509.5	554.4	600.0	645.9	742.0	971.4	1,407.8
Medicare	148.4	266.3	283.8	309.0	335.5	420.1	536.0	792.0
Medicaid[c]	76.8	147.3	162.5	173.1	181.5	184.0	258.9	384.4
Other federal[d]	52.5	95.8	108.1	118.0	128.9	137.8	176.5	231.3
State and local	124.7	217.1	229.0	247.3	268.7	279.2	371.2	519.4
Medicaid[c]	45.6	101.7	108.7	119.6	133.6	136.0	191.5	285.3
Other state and local[d]	79.1	115.4	120.3	127.7	135.0	143.2	179.7	234.1

Average annual growth (percent)	1993[e]	2002	2003	2004	2005[b]	2006[b]	2010[b]	2015[b]
NHE	11.5	6.4	8.2	7.9	7.4	7.3	7.4	7.0
Private funds	11.0	6.2	8.6	7.6	6.9	4.3	7.7	6.5
Consumer payments	11.0	6.2	8.7	7.8	6.8	3.8	7.7	6.4
Out-of-pocket payments	8.0	4.2	6.0	5.5	5.6	–1.0	6.5	5.9
Private health insurance	13.7	7.1	9.8	8.6	7.3	5.5	8.1	6.5
Other private funds	11.1	5.7	7.7	6.8	7.4	7.5	7.6	7.2
Public funds	12.2	6.8	7.8	8.2	7.9	11.0	7.1	7.5
Federal	12.7	7.0	8.8	8.2	7.7	14.9	7.0	7.7
Medicare	13.7	6.7	6.6	8.9	8.6	25.2	6.3	8.1
Medicaid[c]	15.4	7.5	10.3	6.6	4.9	1.4	8.9	8.2
Other federal[d]	9.0	6.9	12.8	9.1	9.2	6.9	6.4	5.6
State and local	11.3	6.4	5.5	8.0	8.7	3.9	7.4	7.0
Medicaid[c]	13.6	9.3	6.9	10.0	11.8	1.8	8.9	8.3
Other state and local[d]	10.4	4.3	4.3	6.1	5.8	6.0	5.8	5.4

Source: Christine Berger and others, "Health Spending Projections through 2015: Changes on the Horizon," *Health Affairs* 25, no. 2, web exclusive (February 22, 2006): W61–W73. Data from Centers for Medicare & Medicaid Services, Office of the Actuary, National Health Statistics Group.

a. Numbers might not add to totals because of rounding. The year 1993 marks the beginning of the shift to managed care. Growth rates are calculated consistent with the methodology of the National Health Expenditure Accounts. For example, the 2015 growth rate above is equal to the level of 2015 expenditures over the level of 2010 expenditures raised to the one-fifth power (the average growth over five years); "2015 growth rate" is shorthand for 2010–15 growth rate. Medicaid spending growth rates are projected to decline from historical trends, yet they remain higher than Medicare and private funds.

b. Projected.

c. Includes Medicaid and State Children's Health Insurance Program (SCHIP) expansion (Title XIX).

d. Includes Medicaid and SCHIP expansion (Title XXI).

e. Average annual growth from 1970 through 1993.

Medicaid expenditures represent 9 percent of the federal budget but 22.9 percent of the typical state's budget and 16.9 percent of the typical state's general fund.[1] Behind these averages exists substantial variation: in Wyoming, Medicaid only consumes 7.7 percent of the state's overall budget, but in Louisiana, Maine, Mississippi, Missouri, Pennsylvania, and Tennessee, it consumes more than 30 percent.

The Centers for Medicare and Medicaid Services (CMS) anticipates that federal Medicaid spending will increase from $181.5 to $384.4 billion over the next ten years, with an annual growth rate of around 8 percent in most years. This is a slight decline from the past but is higher than the forecast for any other payer, including Medicare and private health insurance premiums (table 4-1).

Medicaid's rapid cost growth represents a combination of increased spending per enrollee and an increase in the number of enrollees. Between 2000 and 2003, Medicaid spending increased by one-third, while the cost per enrollee grew at a rate slower than that of private health insurance premiums.[2] Hadley and Holahan concluded that Medicaid costs less than private health insurance on a per-enrollee basis largely because of lower provider payment rates.[3]

Medicaid is a means-tested entitlement program that pays for health care services for 55 million Americans.[4] Medicaid is actually a variety of programs wrapped into one. It provides health care coverage to pregnant women, low-income children, and some poor parents. It pays for long-term care services, including nursing home care and care delivered in the home and community, for frail elders and people with severe disabilities. The program pays for the cost sharing in Medicare that can be unaffordable for poor and near-poor elders. The program is also a source of direct financing to many hospitals that treat large numbers of people without health insurance.

While almost half of Medicaid recipients are children, they account for only 18 percent of program costs (figure 4-1); people with disabilities account for 42 percent of Medicaid spending. This eligibility category is extremely heterogeneous and includes people with severe and persistent mental illness (Medicaid pays for more than a quarter of the nation's spending on mental health services), children with developmental disabilities, people with HIV/AIDS, people with spinal cord injuries, and people with degenerative physical and neurological conditions.[5]

Figure 4-1. *Medicaid Enrollees and Expenditures by Enrollment Group, 2003*

Percent

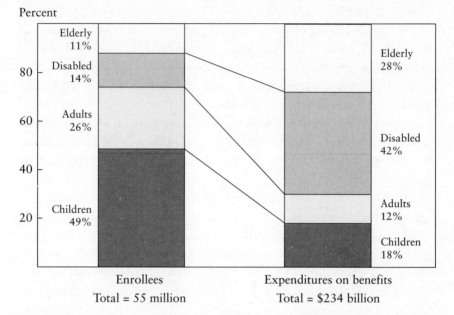

Enrollees   Expenditures on benefits
Total = 55 million   Total = $234 billion

Source: Estimates based on 2003 MSIS data, Urban Institute and Kaiser Commission on Medicaid and the Uninsured.

All Medicaid recipients receive a comprehensive set of medical benefits, with some services required by the federal government and others offered at the discretion of the state. States can (and do) set limits on the "amount, duration, and scope" of benefits, meaning, for example, limits on the number of prescriptions that can be filled (amount) or the period of time physical therapy visits will be covered (duration) or the extent to which all types of mental health services will be paid (scope). Under federal law Medicaid provides children a broader set of benefits than it provides adults.

For the frail elderly and people with disabilities, Medicaid is more than a health care program. Nursing home care includes both medical and residential (that is, room and board) services, and people with disabilities may obtain services that are not medical in nature, such as "personal care assistance"—getting out of bed or preparing meals.

Medicaid's Structural Uniqueness

Compared with the other health programs discussed in this volume, Medicaid is unique for five reasons: it has joint state-federal administration, it has means-tested eligibility, its budget has countercyclical components, it is the dominant payer for certain providers, and it generally has low provider payment rates. All of these features need to be considered when attempting to contain program costs.

STATE-FEDERAL ADMINISTRATION. States have day-to-day responsibility for running the program within the constraints of laws and policies set by the federal government. States that wish to operate outside of the established rules can make formal applications to CMS to waive the rules under a number of provisions of the Social Security Act. The broadest waiver authority appears in section 1115, which grants the secretary of health and human services broad (but not unlimited) authority to waive provisions of the law for the purposes of research and demonstration. On the basis of a rule from the Office of Management and Budget, waivers must be cost neutral to the federal government.

The federal government pays for 57 percent of the overall costs of the Medicaid program.[6] The federal share for covered benefits is set by a formula that varies with state median income, with a floor of 50 percent federal participation. Special matching rates exist in certain categories: administrative costs are shared 50:50, and development costs of claims payment systems are 90:10. Special rates also extend to certain services: family planning services receive a 90 percent federal match.

The shared financing and administrative structure is a constant source of tension in the Medicaid program. The federal government and the states clash over which level of government controls program design. More important for the purpose of this book, the structure provides incentives to increase spending in two critical ways. First, states have a strong incentive to define as many state expenditures as possible as "Medicaid" so they can obtain a federal matching payment to offset a portion of the costs. The challenges raised by this incentive are discussed in greater detail below. Second, the marginal cost to either the federal government or a state is less than one dollar for every dollar of services provided, making it easier for either to decide to expand the program than if financing rested entirely at only one of the levels of government. It is important to note that this inflationary tendency offsets a constricting one. When it comes to social benefits, states inherently under-spend because of concerns about becoming a welfare magnet—a state that attracts needy people from states that have lower benefits.

State administration creates important opportunities for program efficiency. States have brought innovations to Medicaid in many areas, including widespread reliance upon managed care, development of consumer-directed care models, employment of disease management programs, experiments with simplification of program administration, and creative efforts to blend public and private coverage. States truly function as laboratories in the Medicaid program, trying out new ideas and disseminating what works. Flexibility permits states to craft programs that are appropriate to their residents' values, the structure of the health care market, and the availability of health care providers. However, the cost of state flexibility is some administrative redundancy and a degree of variation around the country—particularly with respect to eligibility—that is hard to defend given the dominant funding role of the federal government.

MEANS-TESTED ELIGIBILITY. Medicaid eligibility is dependent upon having very low income and (for most eligibility categories) limited financial assets. Given the extremely limited resources of the enrolled population, any change that eliminates covered benefits is likely to translate primarily into forgone use of health care services. Increases in cost sharing that would be considered modest by a commercial population (from $3 to $5 for a prescription) can be a complete impediment to obtaining services (or simply a cost shift to providers who may not even attempt to collect) for a Medicaid population.[7]

The health consequences of these changes are a matter of some debate. The results of the 1987 RAND health insurance experiment suggested that the overall consequences for health status of moderate increases in patient out-of-pocket costs are minimal or nonexistent.[8] But there were negative effects for low-income people, and more recent analyses considering the interaction between types of care (for example, drugs and physician visits) and the impact of cost sharing on adherence to the treatment regimen warn that health consequences can be substantial.[9]

COUNTERCYCLICAL SPENDING. Medicaid's income-based eligibility rules mean that more people become eligible for the program when the economy weakens and worker incomes fall. In addition, as firms become less likely to offer coverage to their employees or expect their employees to pay more, low-wage workers without a realistic option of holding employer-sponsored insurance are more likely to turn to Medicaid, at least for their children (only a small share of the workers themselves are eligible).

These events occur at a point in the economic cycle when federal and state revenues are likely to be falling. Thus Medicaid cost growth caused by enrollment accelerates just as its funding sources are declining. This inherent dynamic ensures that Medicaid will periodically come under substantial pressure as a budget buster. In addition, it means that when political attention focuses on the program the perception of budget growth will be somewhat overstated, since it will reflect a combination of per-person cost growth and unusually high enrollment growth. This phenomenon was most apparent in the early part of this decade.

DOMINANT PAYER. Medicaid is the dominant payer for many of the services it purchases, which creates an opportunity to influence efficiency. The most obvious example is nursing home care: Medicaid finances care for 60 percent of all nursing home residents.[10] But there are other examples as well. Medicaid pays for residential treatment facilities, adult day care, home care aides, and other services or providers closely linked to the specific needs of a subgroup of the Medicaid population. Many of these services and provider types are not covered by other forms of insurance and are not purchased frequently by people without insurance.

This role for Medicaid has a number of implications. From a political perspective, these providers are dependent upon Medicaid for their livelihood, and they can become a formidable lobbying force with respect to their payments. From a practical perspective, it can be difficult to define or determine appropriate payment rates since there may be little or no private market for similar frail, low-income patients that can be used to establish fair rates or that can provide sustainable rates with normal profits.

LOW, ADMINISTRATIVELY ESTABLISHED PROVIDER PAYMENT RATES. Medicaid pays providers using a fee schedule established by each state, although payments made through managed care organizations may differ from the schedule. In addition, for services that have a mix of payers, such as hospital and physician care, Medicaid generally pays below-market rates. It can do this because some providers have little choice but to accept the established rate and because some of its contracting providers have a charitable, tax-exempt mission.

Medicaid's low payment rates discourage providers from participating in the program if they have other options. Hence recipients can face barriers to access, particularly for some specialty services. From the perspective of the program's fiscal health, the implications are that savings cannot be generated through lowering provider payment rates and that Medicaid providers are unlikely to be able to pursue innovations and investments unless they receive or expect to receive an increase in their rates.

How Could Medicaid Spending Be Controlled?

Conceptually, it would be easy to reduce Medicaid spending. Program eligibility could be curtailed or covered services scaled back. These steps could be taken year after year to meet a predefined budget target, and Medicaid would make its contribution to solving the fiscal problems of the country. Yet this would not be a solution at all because it means these costs are shifted either to providers, other payers, or the people the program is intended to cover. Medicaid was created out of recognition that low-income Americans were not gaining the benefits that the health care system has to offer. Mechanically chipping away at Medicaid risks re-creating these problems.

Our goal must be greater efficiency. In this context, efficiency could mean a few different things:

—Medicaid could be redesigned so that beneficiaries attain the same health and functional status while receiving fewer or less intensive services.

—Medicaid could purchase the same health care services at a lower cost (without those costs simply appearing elsewhere).

—People who rely upon Medicaid could have their needs met through other vehicles, such as employer-sponsored health insurance or private insurance for long-term care.

Ultimately, the challenge is to constrain the growth in program spending without denying people the services they need. In this section we discuss four broad categories of policy changes and handicap their potential benefits and costs: changing state incentives, delivery systems, enrollee incentives, and policies designed to reduce demand for the program.

Policies Designed to Change State Incentives

A variety of policy options are available that would increase state incentives to reduce Medicaid program costs. At one extreme is the option of converting the Medicaid program into a block grant to states. A block grant is a lump sum of money determined in advance through a formula. Federal requirements regarding eligibility rules, covered benefits, and provider payment rates could be preserved (which would cause the states to object) or eliminated (which would cause advocates for Medicaid recipients to object).

The obvious benefit of a block grant to the federal government is that it provides complete budget predictability and a simple lever for controlling future spending. State reactions to a block grant depend upon how large the grant is in the first year, what factors are used to increase the grant over time, how much flexibility it actually gives states to modify their programs, how high a priority the states place on meeting the needs of the Medicaid population, and how the states feel about bearing the risk of filling in the gap between the cost of meeting their populations' needs and the amount the federal government gives them to do so. Currently, if Medicaid spending increases for any reason—a change in the overall economy, a new medical technology, a new disease (for example, HIV/AIDS), changes in eligibility, benefits or payments to providers, or a natural disaster (for example, Hurricanes Katrina and Rita)—the federal government shares the cost with the state. But if a state figures out how to save money in the program, both the state and federal government share in the savings. Thus, the incentives for the states to save are not as high as they could be. Under a block grant a state would have strong incentives because it could keep all the savings.

A block grant would almost certainly change state behavior. States have even responded to congressional *debate* over a block grant—they increased their spending in what they thought would be the base year so they could secure a larger grant in the future, but then they slowed spending when the block grant legislation was vetoed by President Clinton.[11]

The Democratic Party's alternative in the mid 1990s to a block grant was a milder version of constraint—the "per capita cap." The per capita cap limits the federal contribution per enrollee to the state, but it ensures continued matching funds for every person enrolled in the program. The proposal has conceptual appeal: states are held faultless against events outside of their control, such as disasters and economic downturns that cause Medicaid enrollment to grow, but they have strong incentives to control spending per capita, which is where they potentially have leverage. Yet the concept suffers in two critical details. First, determining an appropriate growth factor in per capita spending is difficult (imagine projecting your private insurance premium out ten years into the future). Second, because per capita spending is easy to manipulate by cutting benefits, and Democrats did not want to encourage states to cut benefits, the per capita cap proposal limited state flexibility in ways that made it hard for states to imagine that they could operate within the limits.

Over the years policy analysts of varying points of view have proposed a broad range of "swap" proposals. President Reagan proposed to have the federal government assume full responsibility for Medicaid while states financed welfare, food stamps, and other programs.[12] Today governors regret having rejected that offer. Other proposed swaps include giving full responsibility to either the state or federal level of government for the "dual eligibles"—those eligible for both Medicare and Medicaid— while shifting remaining populations to the other level of government. Since a swap means that one level of government bears full financial responsibility for meeting the needs of the population, it creates many of the same financial incentives as a block grant.

The argument for the swap is that shared fiscal responsibility is a recipe for cost shifting and inefficiency, and indeed there is evidence to support this view. Yet, swap proposals always founder on the shoals of budget projections. Neither level of government wants to take on a larger current or expected future fiscal burden. Neither level of government is sufficiently confident that, given full responsibility for a population, it will be able to meet the needs of that population at lower cost.

Ultimately, support for any of these ideas—block grants, per capita caps, and swaps—arises from a simple notion: given greater financial responsibility, states will be more effective at controlling program costs. Advocates of these approaches believe those savings can come from efficiencies; detractors believe they will come from cuts in services to Medicaid enrollees. What is clear is that under any of these alternative structures states will have strong incentives to achieve efficiencies; what is not clear is whether states have the tools necessary to do so. That question is discussed in later sections of this chapter.

Budget caps also raise substantial fairness issues, since they lock in existing interstate inequities with respect to eligibility levels and provider payment rates. With a cap, the governor or legislature of a state operating a limited program cannot obtain new federal funds even if the state wants to modify its program to bring it up to the level that another state already had in place. In addition, it is difficult for the federal government to set rules that prevent states from scaling back on their coverage and using their block grant funds to support other programs.

A primary benefit of budget caps is that they eliminate fiscal gaming— a recurring problem within Medicaid. Fiscal gaming refers to practices states adopt that are intended *primarily* to maximize federal matching revenue to the states, and not to reimburse providers for the costs of delivering medical services to the eligible population. Budget caps eliminate state incentives and opportunities for gaming.

Over the years states have figured out a number of legal mechanisms to pay providers exaggerated rates, obtain federal funds to cover a share of those rates, and use the federal funds to either reimburse the provider or fill the state treasury. The federal reaction to fiscal gaming to date has been to limit the games one by one. The Government Accountability Office (GAO) says that, although efforts by Congress and the CMS have narrowed fiscal gaming, it has not been eliminated. GAO's 2004 report on improving federal oversight notes that "states can and do continue to claim excessive federal matching funds, using them for non-Medicaid purposes or to inappropriately increase the federal share of Medicaid program expenditures."[13]

The politics of fiscal gaming is filled with irony. Members of Congress rail against egregious practices but defend the same when they are committed by their own states. When a new state trick is discovered, legislation designed to close the loophole gives a few states extra time (during which they will obtain substantial federal dollars) to come into compliance. CMS administrators complain of state practices but do not propose regulations that would control them. Meanwhile, states can make garden-variety excessive or inefficient payments to providers without bumping up against any federal rules or attracting any notice.[14]

Some amount of fiscal gaming may be the price of a matched financing structure. Block grants and caps offer one way out, but so does a more coherent approach targeted specifically at the problem. A recent paper from the National Academy for State Health Policy describes a series of structural steps that could more clearly define what revenue sources can be used to serve as the state match and what types of expenditures are eligible for receiving the federal share.[15] An alternative approach is inspired by Coughlin and Zuckerman who calculated the *effective* federal match percentage (which includes fiscal games) and compared it with the *nominal* federal match percentage derived by federal statutory formula.[16] Rules could be developed so that states with high effective rates relative to their nominal rate would have to repay the difference.

Policies Designed to Change How Care Is Delivered

Within broad federal parameters, each state decides how to operate its Medicaid program, especially with regard to provider participation and payments. States are currently using three levers for improving systems of care for Medicaid enrollees: managed care, disease management, and pay-for-performance, but they could do more.

INCREASED USE OF CAPITATION ARRANGEMENTS FOR MANAGED CARE. A majority of Medicaid recipients are enrolled in managed care plans, and more than thirty states require Medicaid recipients to enroll in such plans. Under Medicaid managed care, health maintenance organizations, prepaid health plans, or comparable entities agree to provide a specific set of services to Medicaid enrollees, in return for a predetermined periodic payment per enrollee. They also agree to follow rules established by the state regarding matters such as the number of physicians, by specialty, who will be available for patient care; quality standards; and patient satisfaction targets. Table 4-2 shows the number of plans and enrollees in Medicaid managed care.

One policy approach is to further encourage growth in Medicaid managed care. Growth in Medicaid managed care has slowed because the easiest and lowest cost groups to enroll, women and children, have largely been enrolled. The more costly and higher-risk disabled have yet to be confronted by most states. Nonetheless, the earliest Medicaid managed care demonstrations documented savings of 5 percent for children and

Table 4-2. *Medicaid Managed Care Plans*[a]

Managed Cared Entity Type	Number of Plans	Number of Enrollees
Health insuring organization	5	500,780
Commercial managed care organization	157	9,780,823
Medicaid-only managed care organization	130	8,606,164
Primary care case management	36	6,559,561
Prepaid inpatient health plan	107	8,119,325
Prepaid ambulatory health plan	43	4,986,161
Program of All-Inclusive Care for the Elderly	33	11,824
Other	8	549,358
Total	519	39,113,996

Source: "Summary Statistics as of June 30, 2005" in *Medicaid Managed Care Enrollment Report* (Department of Health and Human Services, Centers for Medicare & Medicaid Services, Finance, System and Budget Group.

a. This table provides duplicated figures by plan type. The total number of enrollees includes 10,538,411 individuals who were enrolled in more than one managed care plan. It also includes individuals enrolled in state health care reform programs that expand eligibility beyond traditional Medicaid eligibility standards.

adults, and studies of individual states have continued to demonstrate the value of managed versus unmanaged care especially for this population.[17] The savings to be expected from Medicaid managed care for the disabled and dual eligibles, largely the remaining group in unbridled fee-for-service, are less well documented, although the potential yields are greater given the higher cost of this population.

The hopes for managed care must be kept in perspective. The traditional managed care model that has served Medicaid reasonably well with respect to low-income families and children faces new challenges when applied to the more complex needs of people with disabilities and frail elders. The Arizona Health Care Cost Containment System (AHCCCS), which has all Medicaid eligibles enrolled in managed care including for long-term care services, has been in operation more than twenty years. The Program of All-Inclusive Care for the Elderly (PACE) has been in operation for more than fifteen years and was converted to a permanent feature of Medicaid in 2005. Many states have successfully used risk-adjusted managed care payments for their disabled populations. And a number of states have developed capitated payment models for people with mental disabilities. Some states have well-established managed care organizations with experience in enrolling the disabled and frail elderly. Yet most states are on a steep learning curve for further development.

Managed care is particularly difficult to implement in rural areas. There is a sense that Medicaid managed care has succeeded in reaching the goal of predictable, moderate spending growth with reasonable quality of care for most states; yet the growth in managed care has stalled.[18] Supplemental grants, such as PACE grants in 2005, and marginal increases in federal matching rates to encourage states to expand Medicaid managed care might restart the growth in such programs.

DISEASE MANAGEMENT AND ITS VARIANTS. What cost containment strategies are available for those not enrolled in managed care, who are primarily the elderly and disabled poor? It is an important question for Medicaid, because despite the prevalence of managed care, payments to managed care organizations constitute only 15.6 percent of total program spending.[19]

One possible solution is disease management. Disease management is a system of coordinated health care interventions and communications for populations with chronic disease. Patient self-care efforts are a significant aspect of disease management programs because they intervene with physicians, patients, and caregivers to encourage adherence to established medical treatment guidelines for improved outcomes and lower spending.

The idea is not new to Medicaid; it is just poorly dispersed among the states in any standard format. Managed care companies, especially health maintenance organizations, have used disease management programs on behalf of Medicaid recipients for more than thirty years. More than twenty states have disease management programs for adult Medicaid recipients with chronic conditions such as asthma, diabetes, and congestive heart failure. They make a great deal of sense for state Medicaid programs because they have been shown to decrease inpatient and emergency room costs, increase pharmacy costs in accordance with medical treatment guidelines, and produce a net decline in total spending of 3 to 5 percent for the patients enrolled in disease management.[20]

Managed care organizations develop and operate disease management programs on their own as part of their overall care management approach. The fee-for-service portion of Medicaid programs could benefit from well-constructed disease management programs paired with intensive case management for very high cost recipients. Medicaid directors need better information regarding the relative effectiveness of various approaches, as they have legitimately grown skeptical over time of claims that every new thing will save them money. Medicaid disease management programs that support Medicaid providers should have the greatest potential, because they help providers identify patients most in need of assistance, to adopt evidence-based practice guidelines, and report or give feedback routinely about progress in terms of appropriate health care or reasonable costs.

PAY-FOR-PERFORMANCE AND ITS VARIANTS. Traditional fee-for-service inherently rewards the volume of services provided and not necessarily quality and efficiency. By discriminating among providers on the basis of quality and efficiency (and in some cases publishing the results), public and private purchasers might be able to encourage and reward performance improvement efforts. Whether paying for better quality on the margin can help the fiscal crisis in health care is unknown.

Except for a few Medicaid managed care companies in ten states, pay-for-performance is virtually untried in fee-for-service Medicaid. North Carolina has a program with financial rewards and recognition for the above-average primary care physicians who meet minimal process measures for case management of asthma and diabetes and the use of generic medicines. Pennsylvania is making payments to acute care hospitals in the state if they reduce the seven-day readmission rate for certain conditions and reduce the time between diagnosis of pneumonia and treatment with antibiotics. The leader in using pay-for-performance methods, with at least a toe in the water, has been Medicare. With $7 million to $21 million on the line, Medicare has preliminary results from the Premier Hospital demonstration that show improvement in basic process measures of quality among 270 participating hospitals.[21]

Efforts to adopt pay-for-performance in Medicaid will face some hurdles not experienced by Medicare. The primary hurdle is market power. Medicaid may not command attention from providers the way Medicare does. Another hurdle is the ability to analyze and act on available claims data. Medicare has better data than do most Medicaid programs. Smaller states especially lack the infrastructure and sufficient data to go beyond the most basic information systems. Medicaid also suffers from low payment rates and a relatively high concentration of its recipients served by a limited number of already overly stretched providers.

Rewarding performance at the margin may do little to change behavior if providers do not consider themselves appropriately compensated to begin with.

In principle, better quality care should cost less, with fewer costly errors, better care outcomes, and more satisfied patients. In the same way, the performance that is measured and rewarded is usually the only aspect of care that changes. A recent report laments the lack of uniformity in measures of performance and the current coarse state of quality measures that seem to only scratch the surface of performance.[22] Great anticipation is also placed in posting the comparative results of performance measurements of providers so that patients can discern differences in quality measures and vote with their feet for better quality of care. Policymakers and analysts are still learning about the effects of such consumer-directed health care, but a system of care that values the demands of patients, even low-income patients with chronic disease, would surely be superior to one that patronizes them.

Five large states (New York, California, Texas, Pennsylvania, Florida) account for more than 40 percent of total Medicaid spending.[23] If they could begin to develop measurable performance standards in fee-for-service Medicaid and show that they have had an impact on quality and cost, then other states might be able to follow.

Policies Designed to Change the Behavior of Individual Beneficiaries

Since its inception, Medicaid has been a defined benefits plan. This means that certain services, discussed earlier, must be provided by each state to receive federal financial participation, and states can add other specified benefits as they wish. New flexibility offered by the 2005 Deficit Reduction Act has prompted several states, with more to follow, to move away from defined benefits to defined contributions. A defined contribution plan does not promise a set of benefits, rather it promises a payment toward benefits. In many ways, this is bringing Medicaid into alignment with similar trends in private-sector health plans and certain components of Medicare (Part C and Part D).

Two primary models are emerging. One is the direct purchase model, whereby the state gives each Medicaid beneficiary a fixed sum of money that he or she can use to purchase insurance coverage in the private market. A related, much more limited approach is the cash and counseling model, in which Medicaid recipients have the ability to hire, fire, and schedule their personal care services rather than work through a home health agency. The other model is the "rewards" approach for pursuit of healthy behaviors and "penalties" for failing to do so.

VOUCHERS AND VARIOUS DEFINED CONTRIBUTION APPROACHES. Florida typifies the defined contribution approach. It is assigning Medicaid recipients, in different parts of the state, to a risk-adjusted premium for the purchase of insurance from among a selection of state-approved, actuarially equivalent products, each offering different services. The approach has some features in common with the Federal Employee Health Benefits Program, in that those covered receive a fixed subsidy and the plans can vary the benefits.

Milligan, Woodcock, and Burton issued warnings about this approach. They recommended that states ensure that the risk adjustment is accurate and that vital services be grafted onto the defined benefit plans, if necessary.[24] With greater personal responsibility in their hands, Medicaid recipients may need a different set of consumer protections than is normally provided, and state agencies, including the insurance commission, may have to modify their normal way of doing business. Supports should be in place to help Medicaid recipients make informed choices about their health plan, primary provider, and prevention and screening services. Nevertheless, with attentive oversight and quick modification to likely pitfalls, the defined contribution approach could help Medicaid control spending and would give a new generation of recipients the type of coverage that the rest of the covered population has (with all of the advantages and disadvantages that such coverage entails).

FINANCIAL INCENTIVES FOR HEALTH-PROMOTING BEHAVIORS. West Virginia is taking a different approach by requiring eligible recipients to sign a member agreement. By signing the agreement, the Medicaid recipient promises to keep appointments with physicians, adhere to the treatment regimen in terms of taking drugs, and not overuse the hospital emergency room. Failure to keep appointments or to take drugs and unnecessary emergency room visits are three long-standing negative characteristics of any Medicaid program and known to be a source of unnecessary Medicaid spending. Those eligible for Medicaid who refuse to sign or are noncompliant with the agreement will see a reduction in their benefits. They will either face higher cost sharing or find the amount, duration, or scope of benefits curtailed.

Private-sector employers have successfully implemented carrot-and-stick programs for weight control, smoking cessation, and prescription drug adherence.[25] Many state policymakers, frustrated by jammed emergency departments and the combination of rising drug budgets and rising incidence of chronic disease, believe a change is needed in the way Medicaid recipients participate in the program. Certainly, asking the Medicaid recipient to join the team providing the care cannot hurt. What is not yet clear is whether the criteria for obtaining "carrots" can be well defined (physicians have expressed concerns about becoming enforcers on behalf of the state) and what the health consequences will be for those who end up with fewer benefits because of "sticks." The jury is still out on this development, but it bears careful watching for its potential for moderating the rise in Medicaid spending.

Policies Designed to Reduce Demand for the Program

States view Medicaid as an essential part of their current strategies to provide insurance to their low-income populations, cover the chronic care needs of people with disabilities and the elderly, and finance the health care safety net. Medicaid has accomplished much, and it can continue to do so if the underlying fiscal pressures and tensions built into it are addressed.[26] One way to address these pressures is to identify opportunities for other programs or systems to bear some of the burden that Medicaid currently carries. Three ideas that might reduce demand are private insurance for long-term care, premium assistance programs, and a new national eligibility standard paired with dedicated funding.

PROMOTING PRIVATE INSURANCE FOR LONG-TERM CARE. Approximately 17 percent of Medicaid spending nationwide is for nursing home care and an additional 5 percent is for home- and community-based services that enable people to live at home or in less restrictive environments.[27] The rising cost of long-term care, shortages of qualified caregivers in any setting, and the demands stemming from living longer portend major problems for states and their Medicaid budgets, as well as for the federal government.

Private long-term care insurance has been suggested as a partial response. The data are not current, but estimates are that somewhere between 29 and 38 percent of purchasers of long-term care insurance who use nursing homes would qualify for Medicaid payments if they did not own a policy. This is equivalent to between 13 and 17 percent of all policyholders.[28] If the group could be expanded, that is, the number of people with private long-term care insurance could be made larger, especially at the lower end of income, future state spending on Medicaid would be moderated because the private insurance would be the primary payer.

One of the longest-standing approaches to encouraging the purchase of private long-term care insurance is so-called partnership programs, established in 1987 in four states—Connecticut, California, New York, and Indiana.[29] The partnership programs are structured so that purchasers of private long-term care insurance are guaranteed asset protection equal to the costs borne by their insurance. This stands in contrast to what happens in general to people who require long-term care services provided by Medicaid—the state has the obligation to recover its costs from the person's estate when they die. The hope is that the partnership programs will serve as a strong incentive for people to purchase private insurance for long-term care.

There are three barriers to calculating the fiscal impact of the partnership programs. The first barrier is determining the share of people who participate in the partnership programs who would have purchased private long-term care insurance even if the program had not been in place. If this share is large, the public subsidy is simply crowding out a private expenditure that would have been made anyway.

The second barrier is determining the relationship between asset protection in the partnership programs and estate recovery through Medicaid. While federal law requires states to pursue the estates of Medicaid recipients to recover the costs of serving them, most states are not particularly aggressive in this area (reflecting the same aversion to estate taxes expressed by many in the federal government). The partnership program only creates an incentive to purchase coverage if people feel that there is a realistic chance their estate will be held liable, but if that occurs, the cost to the state of providing Medicaid services is reduced by the amount recovered.

The third barrier is determining whether or not, years after purchasing long-term care insurance, people will exhaust their private insurance coverage. If that happens, they become a fiscal burden to Medicaid despite the existence of private coverage, and there are fewer savings for states. It takes a very long time to determine the answer with any assurance. Even so, the GAO found that after nearly 20 years only 251 policyholders in all four of the participating states had exhausted their long-term care insurance benefits.

Largely because of the GAO review of partnership programs, Congress in 2005 lifted the cap on the number of states that can have them, and half the states are now considering them.[30] A nationwide expansion of these programs with new types of long-term products could substantially expand the market for private insurance for long-term care. What is less clear is whether a larger market for long-term care insurance will translate into meaningful savings for the Medicaid program. Some commentators remain skeptical.[31]

PREMIUM ASSISTANCE. More than a dozen states are using Medicaid dollars to help pay the employee's share of the premium in their employer's health insurance plan.[32] These programs, known as premium assistance, have strong conceptual appeal despite limited success in the real world. After years of states' experiments in leveraging Medicaid with private employers, no state has found the right combination of administrative simplification, cost-conscious benefit structure, and affordable premiums to replicate a workable model in other states.[33]

Premium assistance programs face a series of barriers: the limited number of poor people who have an offer of coverage at the workplace, the limited willingness of (particularly small) employers to make any effort to assist with program administration, and the difficulty of supplementing what are often inadequate benefits to meet the more substantial needs of Medicaid enrollees. Nevertheless, states continue their efforts to combine Medicaid coverage with private coverage for low-income persons who work, with the goal of shoring up private coverage while relieving the burden on the taxpayer.

NATIONAL ELIGIBILITY STANDARDS AND NEW FEDERAL FINANC-
ING SOURCES. The politics of Medicaid is a source of strength and a barrier to reform. Changes in Medicaid at the state level are frequently laced
with discussions about what other states are doing, especially neighbor-
ing states. Governors and legislators believe that on the margin low-
income persons will shop for benefits, especially people with serious
disabilities who find that they can get superior coverage in one state versus another or that the eligibility requirements are stricter in one than in
another. One would think this attitude would produce increasing uniformity, but much diversity remains. Any talk in Washington about changing the basic formula for federal financial participation is met with lists
of winning and losing states that always derails any serious discussion
about change.

As difficult as it might be, some have suggested the time has come to
dramatically change the federal-state partnership for the uninsured and
long-term care.[34] The centerpiece of the reform ideas is to establish
national eligibility standards, based on financial need (rather than cate-
gorical eligibility). This would eliminate the disparities across the states in
terms of eligibility and make the program simpler to administer. Accom-
panying this idea is a suggestion that all the states institute reinsurance for
high-risk populations. A prominent feature of the state-run reinsurance
program would be a statewide review of medical necessity and perhaps
even rate setting for high-cost individuals to moderate spending at the
high-cost end of health care.

On the financing side, the federal government could offer Medicaid-
related tax credits to those employers buying into a Medicaid private
managed care plan for their eligible employees. Such a federal tax credit
would help the states' fiscal situation by sharing the costs of Medicaid
coverage, and states could further add their own tax credit for participating employers if they wished to do so.

Renaming Medicaid obviously does not reduce the burden on the state
and federal treasuries. Yet a complete overhaul that simplified the program, increased the investment in care management for those with the
highest costs, and created a new funding stream to support the program
would temper the recurring cries for reform.

How Can Medicaid Contribute to System-Wide Approaches to Control Health Spending?

In Chapter 2, Antos and Rivlin describe a strategy for controlling health spending that blends regulatory and market-based components. They also note the leadership role that federal programs can play in making the strategy work. Medicaid can contribute to the success of this strategy, but the particular needs of the Medicaid population should also be considered as the strategy unfolds.

Medicaid can contribute to efforts to improve the pricing of health care services—particularly paying for performance (P4P). As noted above, a few Medicaid programs are experimenting in this realm, and the lessons they are learning can contribute to the overall body of knowledge on this subject. It is important to note, however, that Medicaid enters the P4P field with rates that are substantially below market. A system-wide effort to improve how the health care system prices services would include raising Medicaid payment rates for many providers. This would have clear negative consequences for the federal and state treasuries, but this increase of payment rates would improve access to care for Medicaid enrollees, with some of this improved access translating into longer-term savings for the program.

Medicaid has been a bit of a latecomer to the health information technology movement.[35] Unlike Medicare, which as a national program has a national claims database, Medicaid administrative data are scattered around the country, and only recently has CMS had any success creating a national Medicaid database. Over time Medicaid should have a great deal to contribute to cost-effectiveness analyses since the program is the dominant payer for such a large share of the population with serious disabilities and chronic conditions.

Medicaid has been at the forefront of developing innovative care models for particular populations served by the program, such as people with HIV/AIDS or traumatic brain injury. Yet dissemination of these models across the states has been spotty, and communication between Medicaid and private insurers on lessons learned has been inadequate. Meanwhile long-noted problems coordinating services for people covered by both Medicaid and Medicare (the dual eligibles) may be overcome in part by the new provisions concerning Special Needs Plans in the Medicare Modernization Act of 2003, although that story has not yet been written. Under the Medicare Modernization Act of 2003 (section 231), Congress created a new type of Medicare Advantage coordinated care plan focused on individuals with special needs. Special needs individuals were identified by Congress as individuals who are institutionalized, are dually eligible, or have severe or disabling chronic conditions.

Engaging the Medicaid enrollee as a consumer raises high hopes and serious cautions. On the one hand, Medicaid's entitlement structure has emphasized the passive role of the enrollee as recipient of services. Efforts to engage Medicaid enrollees in managing their own care and their own health seem appropriate—indeed, Medicaid enrollees with disabilities were at the forefront of the consumer empowerment movement. Yet one must always keep in mind the extremely limited financial resources available to Medicaid enrollees. Levels of cost sharing that might cause a middle-class insured patient to think twice before using a service can present an insurmountable barrier to someone on Medicaid. Financial incentives must be used with great caution in the Medicaid program.

Conclusion

Comprehensive approaches that address the high cost of and inefficiencies in the health care system as a whole offer a way out of the "Medicaid as budget buster" dilemma. Rather than attempting to isolate Medicaid from the rest of the health care system and fix it, decision makers should acknowledge the critical role that Medicaid plays in the health care system and use it as a tool for improving the system as a whole.

Medicaid's experience serving a high-need population can help the overall health care system understand the needs of those with the most expensive health conditions. As analysts have come to understand the critical role chronic conditions play in driving health care costs, Medicaid's experience with these conditions could support improvements in patient care in the population as a whole.[36]

By contrast, attempting to control Medicaid spending without addressing the shortcomings of the health care system as a whole creates a serious risk that the most vulnerable Americans will bear the burden of fiscal controls even as they are the group least able to absorb that burden without negative consequences. There is plenty of room for improvement within the Medicaid program, and improvements must be pursued, but Medicaid cannot solve the nation's fiscal or health system challenges alone.

Medicaid's contribution to the nation's fiscal challenges stems in large part from its role as the nation's safety net. The combination of rising health care costs, increased incidence of disability and chronic disease, and declining private coverage causes more people to drop into that net. And the more the net has to carry, the more it is seen as separate from the mainstream health care system and a welfare program whose costs need to be controlled. If our nation achieved health insurance coverage for everyone, Medicaid's financing challenges would be more similar to those facing the rest of the health care system, and its possible contribution to containing overall health care costs would be more apparent. That should certainly be our goal.

Notes

1. National Association of State Budget Officers, *Fiscal Year 2005 State Expenditure Report* (Washington, Fall 2006).

2. John Holahan and Arunabh Ghosh, "Understanding the Recent Growth in Medicaid Spending: 2000-2003," *Health Affairs* web exclusive, January 26, 2005: W52–W65.

3. Jack Hadley and John Holahan, "Is Health Care Spending Higher under Medicaid or Private Insurance?" *Inquiry* 40, no. 4 (Winter 2003-2004): 323–42.

4. For further information on Medicaid and the State Children's Health Insurance program, see Henry J. Kaiser Family Foundation, "Medicaid and SCHIP" (www.kff.org/Medicaid/index.cfm).

5. Richard G. Frank and Sherry Glied, "Changes In Mental Health Financing Since 1971: Implications for Policymakers and Patients," *Health Affairs* 25, no. 3 (May-June 2006): 601–13.

6. Kaiser Commission on Medicaid and the Uninsured, "The Medicaid Program at a Glance," Fact Sheet 7235 (Washington: Henry J. Kaiser Family Foundation, May 2006) (www.kff.org/medicaid/upload/7235.pdf).

7. Bill J. Wright and others, "The Impact of Increased Cost Sharing on Medicaid Enrollees," *Health Affairs* 24, no. 4 (July-August 2005): 1106–116.

8. Willard G. Manning and others, "Health Insurance and the Demand for Medical Care: Evidence from a Randomized Experiment," *American Economic Review* 77, no. 3 (June 1987): 251–77.

9. Willard G. Manning and others, "Health Insurance and the Demand for Medical Care: Evidence from a Randomized Experiment"; Joseph P. Newhouse, "Reconsidering the Moral Hazard-Risk Avoidance Tradeoff," *Journal of Health Economics* 25, no. 5 (September 2006): 1005–114; John Hsu and others, "Unintended Consequences of Caps on Medicare Drug Benefits," *New England Journal of Medicine* 354, no. 22 (June 1, 2006): 2349–359.

10. Kaiser Commission on Medicaid and the Uninsured, "The Medicaid Program at a Glance."

11. John D. Klemm, "Medicaid Spending: A Brief History," *Health Care Financing Review* 22, no. 1 (Fall 2000): 105–12.

12. Lynn Etheridge, "Reagan, Congress and Health Spending," *Health Affairs* 2, no. 1 (Spring 1983): 15–24.

13. U.S. General Accounting Office, *Medicaid: Improved Federal Oversight of State Financing Schemes Is Needed,* Report to the Committee on Finance, U.S. Senate (Washington: GAO, now named the Government Accountability Office, February 2004) (www.gao.gov/new.items/d04228.pdf).

14. Michael Bond, *Reforming Medicaid,* Policy Report 257 (Washington: National Center for Policy Analysis, 2003) (www.ncpa.org/pub/st/st257).

15. Sonya Schwartz, Shelley Gehshan, Alan Weil, and Alice Lam, "Moving beyond the Tug of War: Improving Medicaid Fiscal Integrity" (Portland, Me.: National Academy for State Health Policy, August 2006).

16. Teresa A. Coughlin and Stephen Zuckerman, "States' Use of Medicaid Maximization Strategies to Tap Federal Revenues," Discussion Paper 02-09 (Washington: Urban Institute, June 1, 2002) (www.urban.org/url.cfm?ID= 310525).

17. Deborah A. Freund and others, "Evaluation of the Medicaid Competition Demonstrations," *Health Care Financing Review* 11, no. 2 (Winter 1989): 81–97.

18. Robert Hurley and Sheldon Retchin, "Medicare and Medicaid Managed Care: A Tale of Two Trajectories," *American Journal of Managed Care* 12, no. 1 (January 2006): 40–44; Robert Hurley and Stephen A. Somers, "Medicaid and Managed Care: A Lasting Relationship?" *Health Affairs* 22, no. 1 (January-February 2003): 77–88.

19. Kaiser Commission on Medicaid and the Uninsured, "The Medicaid Program at a Glance."

20. Louis F. Rossiter and others, "The Impact of Disease Management on Outcomes and Cost of Care: A Study of Low-Income Asthma Patients," *Inquiry* 37, no. 2 (Summer 2000): 188–202; Kenneth Patrick and others, "Diabetes Disease Management in Medicaid Managed Care: A Program Evaluation," *Disease Management* 9, no. 3 (June 2006): 144–56.

21. Centers for Medicare & Medicaid Services, "Medicare Pay-for-Performance Demonstration Shows Significant Quality of Care Improvement at Participating Hospitals," press release, May 3, 2005 (www.cms.hhs.gov/apps/media/press/release.asp?Counter=1441).

22. Institute of Medicine, Committee on Redesigning Health Insurance Performance Measures, Payment, and Performance Improvement Programs, *Performance*

Measurement: Accelerating Improvement (Washington: National Academies Press, 2006).

23. Calculations come from Henry J. Kaiser Family Foundation, "State Medicaid Fact Sheets" (www.kff.org/mfs/index.jsp?CFID=3234822&CFTOKEN=85265301).

24. Charles Milligan, Cynthia Woodcock, and Alice Burton, "Turning Medicaid Beneficiaries into Purchasers of Health Care" (Washington: AcademyHealth, January 2006).

25. John E. Reidel and others, "The Effect of Disease Prevention and Health Promotion on Workplace Productivity: A Literature Review," *American Journal of Health Promotion* 15, no. 3 (Janauary-February 2001): 167–91.

26. Alan Weil, "There Is Something about Medicaid," *Health Affairs* 22, no. 1 (2003): 13–30.

27. Calculations from Centers for Medicare & Medicaid Services, Office of the Actuary, National Health Statistics Group, "National Health Expenditure Data," table 11, "Expenditures for Health Services and Supplies under Public Programs, by Type of Expenditure and Program, Calendar Year 2004" (www.cms.hhs.gov/NationalHealthExpendData/downloads/tables.pdf).

28. Marc A. Cohen, Nanda Kumar, and Stanley S. Wallack, "Long-Term Care Insurance and Medicaid," *Health Affairs* 13, no.4 (Fall 1994): 127–39.

29. U.S. Government Accountability Office (GAO), "The Long-Term Care Partnership Program: An Overview," GAO-05-1021R (September 9, 2005).

30. Vernon Smith and others, "Low Medicaid Spending Growth Amid Rebounding State Revenues: Results from a 50-State Medicaid Budget Survey, State Fiscal Years 2006 and 2007" (Washington: Kaiser Commission on Medicaid and the Uninsured, October 2006).

31. See, for example, Jeffrey Crowley, "Medicaid Long-Term Services Reforms in the Deficit Reduction Act," Issue Paper 7486 (Washington: Kaiser Commission on Medicaid and the Uninsured, April 2006).

32. Information on premium assistance programs is available at www.patoolbox.org.

33. Alice Burton and others, "State of the States: Finding Their Own Way" (Washington: AcademyHealth, January 2006).

34. Lynn Etheredge and Judith Moore, "A New Medicaid Program," *Health Affairs* web exclusive, August 27, 2003: W3-426–W3-439.

35. See Avalere Health, "Evolution of State Health Information Exchange: A Study of Vision, Strategy, and Progress," Publication 06-0057 J (Rockville, Md.: Agency for Healthcare Research and Quality, January 2006).

36. Kenneth E. Thorpe, "The Rise In Health Care Spending And What To Do About It," *Health Affairs* 24, no. 6 (November-December 2005): 1436–445.

5

Leveraging Other Federal Health Systems

SUSAN D. HOSEK

The Veterans Health Administration (VHA) and Military Health System (MHS) are the two largest federal health programs directly providing health care in federally owned and operated hospitals and clinics.[1] In fiscal year 2006, they will spend about $70 billion on health care for approximately 16 million enrolled veterans and active duty and retired military personnel and their beneficiaries.[2] With about one-tenth of the budget of Medicaid and Medicare, the health systems for veterans and the military are small compared to those programs. Controlling their future costs will have little effect on the total federal health care budget.

Nevertheless, these federal health systems can play a larger role in health care reform than their size might suggest. Previous chapters pointed to evidence that federal (and private-sector) health care dollars are not buying consistently high quality care. Improving the value of public and private health spending will require a focus on both efficiency and quality of care. VHA and MHS can be innovative and can set an example for the rest of the U.S. health sector because they are integrated systems that both pay for and, to a considerable extent, provide care and because they are not bound by the myriad constraints in state health regulation. In some areas—including electronic medical records, pharmaceutical costs, and quality-of-care improvement—one or both systems have been leaders. In other areas, they could be more innovative.

Although VHA and MHS account for a small fraction of total federal health care spending, rising spending is of considerable concern to the Department of Veterans Affairs (VA), Department of Defense (DoD), and their constituencies. The scope of benefits provided to veterans' and military beneficiaries has grown over time, and today the benefit packages are significantly better than the benefits available in almost all private employer health plans. As a result, potential beneficiaries increasingly want to take advantage of these relatively generous benefits, and Congress has significantly expanded eligibility for both programs. More eligible beneficiaries are using the systems, and more are dropping their employer coverage in consequence. The expansion in these populations served may continue well into the future and may drive up spending even faster than spending for the health care system in the United States as a whole.

VA and DoD have sought to control their health care budgets by proposing modest increases in cost sharing and adopting management initiatives from the private sector. The proposed cost-sharing increases were intended to moderate the demand for care by those beneficiaries who already rely on the two systems and to discourage additional eligible beneficiaries from shifting into the systems and out of private coverage. Congress has not supported the proposed increases, however. Higher cost sharing is actively opposed by the veterans and military associations, who can marshal strong public support—especially in wartime. With benefit changes ruled out, VHA and MHS will have to focus on improving the efficiency with which they provide benefits.

Evolution of Veterans' and Military Health Care

Each of the two health care systems was established for a narrowly defined purpose, and each has expanded its scope over time. The origins of the systems date back to the beginning of the United States, when they were established to treat the casualties of successive wars and provide ongoing care for those whose injuries were disabling. Up to World War II, the military maintained only a small medical system to care for active duty personnel in peacetime, while the veterans' system grew from a single facility established in 1811 to a system of fifty-four hospitals in 1930.[3]

After World War II, both systems grew rapidly. DoD kept a much larger peacetime medical establishment to support a large standing armed force countering the perceived Soviet threat in central Europe. In 1995, just after the end of the cold war, MHS operated 130 hospitals and 388 clinics in the United States. This large system provided only a fraction of the medical capacity that the military services estimated they would need for a conventional war in Europe. More recently, the post–cold war drawdown resulted in a smaller system comprising 52 hospitals and 309 clinics in the United States that is more than adequate for military needs.[4]

Following World War II, VA significantly expanded its medical system to handle the many disabled veterans, with the system growing over time to its current size of 171 medical centers and more than 350 clinics.[5] Currently, VA projects a decline of 40 percent in the veteran population in the next three decades; in 2004 the Capital Asset Realignment for Enhanced Services (CARES) Commission proposed facility changes to prepare for future demographic and health care delivery changes.[6]

Expansion of Military Health Care

Within DoD, MHS needed patients to keep its many providers busy in its large postwar peacetime system, so active duty dependents, retirees, and retirees' dependents were provided "space-available" access to care in military treatment facilities (known as MTFs). By this time, the nation's employer-based insurance system was in place, and in 1958 MTF space-available care was supplemented by CHAMPUS, a fee-for-service insurance program that financed care provided in the civilian sector for military beneficiaries under the age of 65.[7] MTF care was free of charge, but CHAMPUS included cost-sharing provisions that were similar to many health insurance plans at the time. CHAMPUS covered services for active duty dependents and retirees and their dependents until the age of 65, when these beneficiaries enrolled in Medicare.

In the mid-1990s the MHS adopted managed care practices and transformed the MTF-CHAMPUS program into a new program called

TRICARE. TRICARE continues the old benefit in an option called Standard, but it adds a preferred provider option (PPO) called Extra and a health maintenance organization (HMO) called Prime. Beneficiaries choose either Standard with Extra or Prime; retirees pay a nominal annual enrollment fee for Prime—$230 for single coverage and $460 for family coverage—but active duty dependents pay no enrollment fee for either option.[8]

In the decade since it was implemented, TRICARE benefits have remained constant or even improved while employer insurance has become significantly less generous. For military retirees, TRICARE cost-sharing provisions have remained constant during the past decade. In 2001 Congress eliminated all cost sharing for active duty dependents enrolled in Prime, except for very modest charges for prescription drugs. More recently, Congress also added new benefits for military retirees aged 65 and older and military reservists.

In the decade that TRICARE has been in existence, the under-65 retired population has gradually shifted out of employer insurance to take advantage of the increasingly generous DoD benefit. As figure 5-1 illustrates, in 2005 over half of these beneficiaries relied exclusively on TRICARE, and 14 percent relied only on civilian insurance.[9] Three-quarters of retirees who were eligible for TRICARE used it in 2005. In addition, the over-65 retired population now makes significant use of its new TRICARE for Life benefit. In contrast, few reservists have enrolled in their new benefit, called TRICARE Reserve Select, because they must pay a sizeable premium.[10] This is the one remaining group still looking for expanded eligibility and a more generous military health benefit.

Expansion of Veterans' Health Care

The veterans' health system was also initially developed for a specific purpose—to care for veterans who were seriously injured or who developed long-term illnesses because of wartime military service.[11] Current VHA eligibility rules give highest priority to those who have a significant "service-connected" disability resulting from their injury or illness. As with the DoD system, need for care by these veterans has varied, and so at times the VA system has had excess capacity. As early as 1924, Congress authorized impoverished veterans to use the system to fill the unused capacity.

Figure 5-1. *Insurance Choices of Military Retirees under the Age of 65*

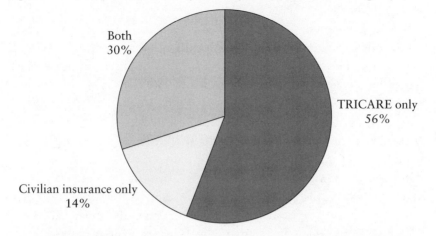

Both
30%

TRICARE only
56%

Civilian insurance only
14%

Source: Louis T. Mariano and colleagues, *Health Insurance Options for Military Retirees under 65: Results from a 2005 Survey,* MG-583-OSD (Santa Monica, Calif.: RAND Corporation, forthcoming).

World War II led to a large expansion of the VA system, initially to provide acute care to veterans and then to specialize in the rehabilitative care veterans needed but could often not get in the civilian sector. Since then, Congress has further expanded VHA eligibility. The Veterans' Health Care Eligibility Reform Act of 1996 made all veterans eligible for the first time; in particular, it authorized access to VHA by veterans who have no service-connected disability or other special circumstance and who are not poor. Veterans must enroll to obtain care, and priority for enrollment is determined by which of eight eligibility categories a veteran falls into. Veterans with major service-connected disabilities have top priority, and nondisabled veterans who exceed an income threshold have lowest priority.

Also like MHS, VHA implemented major changes in the 1990s, responding to the emergence of managed care health systems in the private sector. The VHA was reorganized to incorporate procedures used by managed care organizations and to reflect modern principles of organizational structure.[12] With the management reorganization, VHA reorganized its care delivery system, shifting patients from inpatient to outpatient treatment where possible and opening a network of outpatient clinics in areas previously not served by the VHA.

Unlike TRICARE, the VHA benefit is not strictly an entitlement, even for enrolled veterans. VHA funding is discretionary, and the system is expected under normal circumstances to meet the needs of its enrollees within its budget. The agency is directed by law to "ensure that the provision of care to enrollees is timely and acceptable in quality."[13] Thus the congressional intent is clearly to afford enrollees a benefit that comes close to an entitlement. Consistent with this intent, Congress may choose to supplement the VHA budget, and it did so twice in recent years—in 2002 and 2005. Generally, however, VHA has tried to keep enrollment at a level that the discretionary budget can support. Enrollment of veterans in the lowest priority category was suspended in January 2003 and has not been reopened. Before that date, veterans wanting to enroll faced long delays in some geographic areas, and appointment delays were also common.

The delay and suspension in enrollment is undoubtedly one reason for the difference in reliance of veterans on VHA and military beneficiaries on MHS. Veterans have shifted from private sources of care to the VHA, just as military beneficiaries have. However, only 30 percent of 25 million veterans are enrolled in the system. Almost 80 percent of all veterans have other insurance, including Medicare for roughly one-half of the population. Enrollment rates across priority categories range from 10 to 90 percent, but four-fifths of current enrollees come from priority categories that had access to the system before 1996 (figure 5-2).[14]

Many enrolled veterans get only part of their care from VHA. The most reliant groups—veterans with significant disabilities—get only about half of their care from VHA. In the lowest priority groups, where enrollment is currently frozen, enrollees have an average reliance rate of only 20 percent. Clearly, there is potential for increased use of VHA by all veteran groups if VHA capacity constraints were eased.

Trends in MHS and VHA Users and Budgets

In the decade after Congress enacted eligibility reform in 1996, the number of veterans who enrolled in and used VHA doubled. The largest increases were for category 7 veterans, whose incomes are below the federal levels

Figure 5-2. *Veterans' Reliance on the Veterans Health Administration, 2004*

Percent care from VA

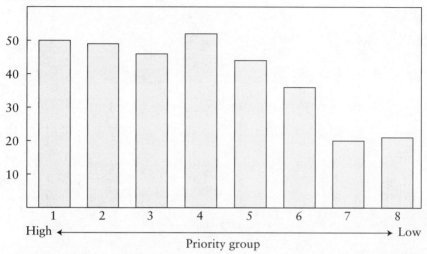

High ← Priority group → Low

Source: Congressional Budget Office, *The Potential Cost of Meeting Demand for Veterans' Health Care* (March 2005), figure 3, p. 7.

for subsidized housing, and those over the age of 65.[15] With some lag, figure 5-3 shows that VHA's budget has kept up with this growth. This crude comparison of total users with the budget suggests that eligibility expansion has been an important factor in recent budget increases. Looking to the future, VHA expects that veterans' utilization of services will continue to increase, in large part because the population is aging. It also expects that the intensity of services provided will increase.[16]

DoD's beneficiary population remained relatively constant throughout the 1990s at roughly 8.5 million, but call-ups of reservists have brought the beneficiary population total to 9.2 million in recent years. DoD's budget growth during the same period was similar to VHA's, with most of the increase occurring after 2000; since then, costs have grown more than 12 percent annually, compared with 8 percent for VHA (figure 5-4).[17] The difference is primarily due to TRICARE for Life, which added $4.6 billion in 2003 and an estimated $7.1 billion in 2006.

Figure 5-3. *Users of Veterans Hospital Administration and Budget,*
1995–2006

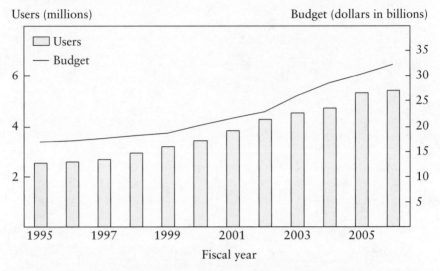

Source: Data from 1995 to 2004 are from Sidath V. Panangala, *Veterans' Medical Care Funding:*
FY1995–FY2004 (Washington: Congressional Research Service, 2005); data for 2005 to 2006 are from
congressional submissions for Medical Programs, tables 3B-2 and 3B-5.

The Congressional Budget Office (CBO) estimates that MHS spending
in 2020 will range from $42 billion to $52 billion in 2002 dollars; the
projected increase in real spending over seventeen years (from the base
year 2003 to 2020) is 2.3 to 3.9 percent per year. CBO's projections for
the VHA budget are in a narrower range; by 2025 the budget is projected
to increase to between $53 billion and $57 billion, reflecting a relatively
low 3.1–3.6 percent annual real rate of growth. Thus the combined budget for military and veterans' health care could grow from about $70 bil-
lion to well over $100 billion in today's dollars in the next 20 years.
However, if general health care spending continues its rapid rise and more
retired beneficiaries shift to TRICARE and VHA, the CBO projections are
likely to be too conservative.[18]

This year, both DoD and the VHA asked Congress to narrow the gap
in cost sharing between their systems and private-sector plans. DoD
requested substantial increases in retiree enrollment fees in TRICARE,
deductibles in the Standard and Extra plans, and pharmacy co-pays. The

Figure 5-4. *Users of the Military Health System and Budget, 1995–2006*[a]

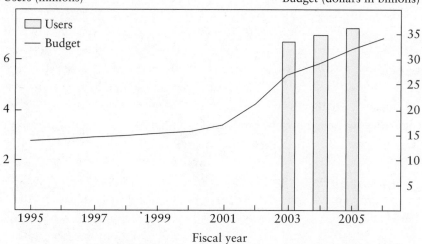

Users (millions)   Budget (dollars in billions)

Source: Author's calculations based on annual reports to Congress on TRICARE. See Department of Defense, TRICARE, Health Program Analysis and Evaluation Division website "Reports" (www.tricare.mil/ocfo/hpae/reports.cfm).
a. 1996–99 budgets are interpolated.

VA requested a modest $250 annual enrollment fee and higher co-pays for prescription drugs, to be paid only by veterans in the two lowest priority categories. Congress did not support these requests. At least while so many military personnel are deployed and at risk in Iraq and elsewhere, both health care systems will find it difficult to increase beneficiary cost sharing. Even in peacetime, there is significant public support for sustaining benefits for military personnel and veterans.

Cost-Effectiveness of Direct Provision of Care by the MHS and VHA

To put MHS and VHA costs in perspective, policymakers would like to know how the costs the systems incur to treat their beneficiaries compare with what the care would cost in the private sector. Is it more or less costly to provide care directly in federal facilities? Further, is direct care more or less effective than care provided in the private sector? For health care, effectiveness is typically thought to encompass several outcomes including access to care, quality of care, and patient satisfaction.

More information for assessing cost-effectiveness is available for VHA than it is for MHS. Nugent and others measured the costs of all health care services provided in six diverse VA facilities in 1999 and estimated what those same services would have cost in the private sector at Medicare prices. They concluded that purchasing the care would have cost at least 20 percent more than providing it directly.[19] Approximately one-half of the difference was attributed to the much lower prices VHA (and MHS) pays for prescription drugs through the Federal Supply Schedule.

A number of recent studies have shown that VHA's quality of care compares favorably with the quality of care provided in the private sector. More than a decade ago, as part of its broader reorganization, VHA established a quality improvement initiative. This initiative apparently has paid off. Asch and others reported that, in a comparison with a matched national sample of patients, VA patients were more likely to receive recommended chronic care and preventive care—the types of care for which VA actively monitors performance—and as likely to receive recommended acute care.[20] Two subsequent studies reached a similar conclusion. Kerr and others found that process of care and intermediate outcomes were better for VHA diabetes patients than those for similar patients in leading managed care organizations.[21] Selim and others concluded that mortality rates were lower in VHA than the rates in Medicare Advantage programs.[22] These studies have established VHA's reputation as a leader in quality-of-care improvement among U.S. health care organizations.[23]

There is less published research that compares cost with quality outcomes in MHS and the private health care system. Goldberg with others compared the costs of all care in the MTF system with what the care would cost if TRICARE purchased it from civilian providers.[24] Similar to the VHA study, the results favor the MTFs. For the median facility, MTF costs were about one-quarter lower; only 15 percent of MTFs had higher costs than facilities of the private sector.

These comparisons of costs in VHA and MHS versus the private health care sector should be viewed with caution for a number of reasons. They are based on very different cost accounting systems and, in the case of

DoD, are based on an allocation of costs between purely military medical support activities and TRICARE activities that is difficult to calculate. The comparisons also hold constant the amount of care provided: for DoD, there is some evidence that more care is provided when beneficiaries use the MTFs than when they use civilian providers.[25] Accurate comparisons of per capita costs cannot be made because most veterans and many TRICARE beneficiaries have dual insurance coverage and because information on the type of care and costs covered by the other insurance is not generally available.

Research on quality of care in the military system comparable to the studies of VHA has not been done. In 1999 responding to news stories about instances of poor care, Congress chartered the DoD Healthcare Quality Initiatives Review Panel to investigate the processes DoD employs to ensure quality. The panel findings included a recommendation to develop data systems that can support measurement of key outcomes including quality. DoD recently announced that it had completed implementation of its electronic medical record system, and studies of quality employing methods similar to the ones applied to VHA data should be possible in the future.

Both VHA and MHS conduct surveys to track patient experiences and satisfaction. DoD reports data from these surveys in its annual report to Congress. Satisfaction improved as TRICARE matured; by 2006, although TRICARE lagged civilian managed care organizations on some measures, the differences were small.[26]

Prospects and Options for Providing Health Care to Veterans and Military Personnel

There is strong political support for seeing to the health care needs of current and former military personnel. Consequently, VHA and MHS now provide a comprehensive set of services at minimal cost to the patient, and the number of beneficiaries who are eligible for and use these services has increased, as other health care sources have become relatively less attractive. The movement of veterans from other health care providers to VHA has been limited by the size of the discretionary budget, which has led to a partial enrollment freeze and queues for appointments. Future

VHA budgets will be determined by congressional decisions about funding greater access to the system. In contrast, TRICARE is an entitlement with open-ended access to purchased care from civilian providers. Most military beneficiaries use MHS for a substantial fraction of their care; in the future, the major source of additional demand is the reserve population. How many reservists switch to TRICARE will depend on whether their premium share remains similar to employer plans. If the reserve benefit is enhanced over time, as the benefit for other military beneficiaries has been, MHS budgets could increase more rapidly than current projections show.

While controlling future costs will make little difference in the overall federal budget picture, within VA and DoD rapidly increasing health spending may constrain budgets for other programs important to their missions. It is worth considering whether providing care directly to the veteran and military populations continues to be cost-effective and what options may be available for controlling future costs. One option, suggested by those who believe public organizations are inherently inefficient, is to outsource VHA and MHS health care services. Another is to modify the benefit to deter switching from employer insurance.

Outsourcing VHA and MHS Care

There are limits to how much and what types of care could be outsourced. VHA has areas of highly specialized expertise that would be hard to match in the private sector. This expertise includes the treatment and rehabilitation of catastrophically injured patients and treatment of certain mental health conditions, including posttraumatic stress disorder.

MHS requires a substantial number of active duty health personnel to support military operations. For the third time in the past fifteen years, DoD is undertaking a major review of its medical personnel requirement. The review is expected to conclude that the requirement remains large but is less than the number of active duty medical personnel MHS currently has in its active duty medical service. The question is whether the marginal cost of a larger-than-required MTF system is less than the cost of purchasing more care from civilian providers. This question has been debated for many years. A major DoD study in the early 1990s concluded that expanding the MTFs beyond the minimum necessary for military purposes is the more costly choice because beneficiaries have higher utilization rates when they use MTFs (largely because the care is free). There are a number of reasons to be cautious about this conclusion. The methodology of this analysis was challenging, the data systems at the time had important limitations, and—most important—the study was conducted before TRICARE.

The published research on VHA and MHS cost-effectiveness, although limited, suggests that outsourcing is not likely to significantly lower costs or improve quality. These two systems appear to pay less for the resources they use to provide services than they would pay to purchase the same services in the private sector. VHA quality compares favorably with quality nationwide; however, no comparable evidence on MHS quality is available. Access to VHA care continues to be below private-sector standards, but access has improved and could be further improved at a cost—including the cost of increased utilization by enrolled veterans who would find it easier to get care.

MHS already purchases one-half of the care provided through its managed care contracts. This fraction has increased over time as the Base Realignment and Closure process has closed military hospitals or turned them into clinics. VHA purchases a limited amount of care only when it cannot be provided in any other way. In the absence of compelling evidence for outsourcing and given the special requirements for these two federal health systems, it appears unlikely that either of them will outsource significantly more care than they do now.

Modifying VHA and MHS Benefits

VHA and MHS health costs have risen rapidly because their beneficiaries increasingly find that they can get good care at much lower cost from these systems than through their employer health plans—if they still have employer coverage.

The most direct option for deterring beneficiary switching is to narrow the gap in premium contributions. The average annual employee contribution in the private sector was $612 for single coverage and $2,712 for family coverage in 2005.[27] Veterans pay nothing to enroll in VHA, and Congress recently rejected a proposed $250 annual contribution for veterans with higher incomes.[28] TRICARE requires a contribution from retirees who elect to enroll in Prime or from reservists, but not otherwise. The annual retiree contributions of $230 for single coverage and $460 for family coverage have not changed since TRICARE was implemented a decade ago.[29] The difference in premium cost between TRICARE and private employer plans will continue to grow over time unless TRICARE premiums are increased, but Congress also rejected a Defense Department proposal to gradually increase retiree premiums to around half the average for employer coverage for retired senior officers and less for other retirees.

Cost sharing for private-sector care in TRICARE is roughly similar to other employer plans. However, there is no charge for care in MTFs or, for most veterans, from VHA. Introducing a co-pay for visits would reduce outpatient utilization, but evidence from private-sector HMOs suggests that overall cost savings are likely to be modest. However, a recent study showed that people are highly responsive to the price they pay for prescriptions.[30] TRICARE charges nothing for prescriptions filled at MTFs and less than typical employer plans for prescriptions filled in their retail pharmacy network or mail-order system. VHA charges many veterans $8 a prescription. Updating prescription co-pays to employer-plan levels would likely lead to noticeable cost savings. To lower the financial impact, the higher co-pays could be waived for some beneficiaries and subjected to an annual cap as VHA already does. Nevertheless, Congress has also been resistant to proposals for increases in pharmacy co-pays.

Given congressional resistance to modest increases in premium contributions or other forms of cost sharing for military personnel and veterans, health care decisionmakers interested in controlling future VHA and MHS spending may need to find some other way to induce beneficiaries to rely on employer and other private insurance to the maximum extent possible.

For example, military retirees might be offered a new benefit option in lieu of TRICARE that would cover premiums and out-of-pocket costs in employer plans. There are other benefits that could be offered to induce these beneficiaries to enroll in and rely on their employer plans—for example, a long-term care benefit, which is not currently a part of the military package. More information is needed to determine whether any of these approaches would realize significant savings, how retirees would react to the idea, and how to design the most cost-effective approach for military personnel and retirees. Given the substantial savings for DoD if under-65 retirees take full advantage of their employer benefits, an investment in information and analysis would appear to be warranted.

It is difficult to identify a benefit that would induce veterans to limit their use of VHA, that would be consistent with a discretionary budget, and that would support the needs of many veteran users. A cash benefit to offset the out-of-pocket costs for employer insurance would inevitably become an entitlement. Further, many of the biggest users of VHA have health care needs that may be difficult to meet in an employer health plan.

In the short run, it is likely that VHA and MHS benefits will remain attractive in comparison with many employer plans. The growth in their budgets will depend critically on whether Congress funds the enrollment of all veterans who want to get care from VHA and keeps the military reserve health benefit comparable with employer benefits.

Leading Improvement in Health Care Cost and Quality

Overall, VHA and MHS are successful public health organizations. They provide care that has been demonstrated or is widely believed to be of high quality at a cost that appears comparable with private-sector costs. Both systems have adopted innovations from the private sector and have been innovators. Several VHA or MHS initiatives demonstrate the ability of both to innovate. These include electronic medical records, coordination of care by different providers, pharmaceutical purchasing, and improvement in quality and patient safety. Other promising ideas for health care reform, such as pay-for-performance for individual providers, have received less attention but may be usefully explored by VHA and MHS.

Electronic Medical Records

Electronic medical records (EMR) have considerable potential for improving care and saving money.[31] However, EMR systems are complex and expensive to develop and require adaptation of medical practice to be fully effective. VHA pioneered in EMR with its Veterans Health Information System and Technology Architecture (VistA) system and its predecessor, which was implemented as long ago as 1985.[32] VistA archives comprehensive diagnostic and treatment information for each patient, accessible to any provider within the same facility. In addition to patient care information, VistA includes financial and management information. Recently, VHA made its system available to private-sector providers at nominal cost. Under the current version of VistA, providers in one facility cannot access EMR information on care provided to their patients in other facilities, but VHA is developing an upgrade that would make a record accessible to all VA providers in the system. Despite its limitations, VistA has provided VHA with the information needed for its exemplary quality improvement program and a functional EMR system that private health care providers can use.[33]

DoD recently announced that it is close to full implementation of its EMR, called the Armed Forces Health Longitudinal Technology Application (AHLTA). AHLTA contains a central record for every MHS patient that is accessible throughout the system, including on the battlefield. Future plans call for connecting the system with private-sector providers in the TRICARE network and, jointly with VHA, building a new medical imaging data system (for example, X-ray).

VHA and MHS experience with EMR is potentially very valuable to the health sector as a whole. Both systems can make important contributions to knowledge of designing a cost-effective system, implementation, training requirements, and methods for exploiting EMR systems for improving health system outcomes such as quality of care, patient safety, provider productivity, and patient service. There are a few studies of VistA, but many more should be done for both EMR systems. Given their differences, comparisons of outcomes under VistA and AHLTA would be instructive.

Coordinating Care by Different Providers

VHA and MHS purchase care for their patients in the private sector; purchased care, however, is a small fraction of the care provided to veterans but a significant fraction for military beneficiaries. Coordinating care provided within and outside the systems has proved to be difficult. In establishing TRICARE, MHS created a process for facilitating the referral of patients between the MTFs and the private sector. VHA is conducting a demonstration project, beginning this year, to develop its own approach to this challenging problem. Four of VHA's regional networks will work with private-sector partners to develop and implement interventions. TRICARE's program was implemented as part of a package of reforms, and an evaluation of this single component was not possible. However, VHA's initiative will be the subject of an independent evaluation.

Pharmaceutical Costs

The VHA negotiates prices for pharmaceutical drugs through the Federal Supply Schedule, and the MHS is able to take advantage of the resulting low prices, which are comparable with those that the Canadian National Health Service pays.[34] However, Federal Supply Schedule prices were higher during a period when they applied to Medicaid as well as VA and DoD, suggesting that significant volume discounting can be negotiated only if the covered population does not become too large.[35] Expanding Federal Supply Schedule purchasing to Medicare and Medicaid would save far less for those programs and increase costs for the VA and DoD.[36]

Quality Improvement and Patient Safety

As discussed above, VHA's achievements in this area have been documented in research using sophisticated methods, whereas there is no similar research for the MHS. Over the past 10 years, the Institute of Medicine has brought national attention to a quality problem in U.S. health care. For most of this period, VHA's Quality Enhancement Research Initiative (QUERI) program has sought to translate evidence-based research on quality into clinical practice improvements. By publishing its evidence-based research and supporting broad assessments of its quality outcomes, QUERI is a model for MHS and other large public health systems as well as the private sector.

Performance Incentives

VHA and MHS have both sought to enhance the performance incentives in their systems. Both have adopted regional management structures with accountability for outcomes; until now, VHA's structure has been clearly superior for this purpose. DoD recently decided not to adopt a unified medical command, but it continues to seek ways to streamline and integrate TRICARE management.[37] As in other areas, researchers have studied

VHA's experience with organizational reform.[38] Given the unusual MHS structure, with four separate management structures for the Army, Navy, and Air Force systems and the TRICARE contracts, less may be learned of relevance to other health systems from studying its organizational effectiveness.

Neither system has so far adopted provider-level incentives for clinical performance, which many believe will be needed to induce physicians to adopt evidence-based improvements in their practice of medicine. VistA and AHLTA can provide the information needed to design and implement performance-based incentives at the individual and group level (including performance-based pay and other incentives). There may be no better place to learn whether these incentives will be effective and how to design them.

Learning from the VHA and MHS Experience

VHA and MHS can lay claim to excellence and innovation in other areas as well. MHS has made great strides in treating combat casualties, developing new technologies that can be applied in other settings. In partnership with the Indian Health Service, the two systems are exploring methods for delivering care in the most remote areas in Alaska. The federal government should ask its two large integrated health systems to continue to aggressively develop and test new approaches and disseminate information about what works and does not work to the broader health care sector. A more systematic and open evaluation of broad VHA and MHS outcomes and new initiatives will lead to improved public accountability and knowledge helpful in improving the nation's health care system.

Finally, the parallel histories of VHA and military health care illustrate some realities of public health benefits. For programs that serve beneficiaries whose welfare is important to the public, Congress finds it easier to expand benefits than to reduce benefits or increase cost sharing, even in nominal terms. When congressional action results in a relatively generous public system that covers employed people, they will be tempted to drop their employer coverage, especially as cost sharing rises under employer-provided plans. In this regard, there are parallels to other federal health programs, including Medicare and Medicaid.

Notes

1. The Indian Health Service (IHS) also provides health care directly, as well as through tribally contracted and operated health programs, and purchases from private providers. It is a much smaller system than the VHA and MHS; it serves 1.8 million American Indians and Alaska Natives with an annual appropriation of approximately $3 billion. See the Indian Health Service website, "Year 2006 Profile" (http://info.ihs.gov/Files/ProfileSheet-June2006.pdf).

2. See U.S. Department of Veterans Affairs, "Medical Programs" in *Fiscal Year 2007 Budget Submission,* Washington, February 2006 (www.va.gov/budget/summary/1514Chapter3B.pdf); U.S. Department of Defense, "The Military Overview Statement," David S. C. Chu, under secretary of defense for personnel and readiness, and William Winkenwerder Jr, assistant secretary of defense for health affairs, testimony before the Senate Committee on Armed Services Subcommittee on Personnel, 109th Cong., 2d sess., April 4, 2006 (www.tricare.mil/planning/congress/downloads/2006/04-04-06SASCChuWinkenwerderOMBFinal.pdf); U.S. Department of Defense, *Evaluation of the TRICARE Program: FY 2006 Report to Congress,* Washington, March 13, 2006 (www.tricare.mil/ocfo/_docs/eval_report_fy06.pdf).

3. Department of Veterans Affairs website, "VA History" (www.va.gov/about_va/vahistory.asp).

4. DoD, *Evaluation of the TRICARE Program: FY 2006 Report to Congress.*

5. "VA History."

6. CARES Commission, *Capital Asset Realignment for Enhanced Services,* Report to the Secretary of Veterans Affairs (Washington: Department of Veterans Affairs, 2004) (www.carescommission.va.gov/cares_charter.asp).

7. CHAMPUS: Civilian Health and Medical Program of the Uniformed Services.

8. Figures available at the Department of Defense TRICARE website, "TRICARE Costs" (www.tricare.mil/tricarecost.cfm).

9. Louis T. Mariano and colleagues, *Health Insurance Options for Military Retirees under 65: Results from a 2005 Survey,* MG-583-OSD (Santa Monica, Calif.: RAND Corporation, forthcoming).

10. The premium for TRICARE Reserve Select enrollment varies from 50 to 85 percent of the cost of the coverage, depending on access to other (for example, employer) insurance. See U.S. Congress, House, *National Defense Authorization Act for Fiscal Year 2006,* HR 1815, 109th Cong., 1st sess. (January 4, 2005), title VII, subtitle A, sec. 702, "Expanded Eligibility of Members of the Selected Reserve under the TRICARE Program" (www.tricare.mil/planning/congress/downloads/2006/PublicLaw109163.pdf).

11. See Sidath V. Panangala, *Veterans' Medical Care Funding: FY1995–FY2004,* CRS Report for Congress (Washington: Library of Congress, Congressional Research Service, January 14, 2005).

12. See Kenneth W. Kizer, *Prescription for Change: The Guiding Principles and Strategic Objectives Underlying the Transformation of the Veterans Healthcare*

System (Washington: Department of Veterans Affairs, March 1996); Department of Veterans Affairs, Office of Inspector General, *Audit of Veterans Integrated Service Network (VISN 10): Organization, Planning, and Implementation of Key Strategic Goals and Objectives,* 9D2-A19-001 (January 12, 1999); Jeff Luck and John W. Peabody, "Improving the Public Sector: Can Reengineering Identify How to Boost Efficiency and Effectiveness at a VA Medical Center?" *Health Care Management Review* 25, no. 2 (Spring 2000): 34–44.

13. Title 38: Veterans' Benefits, pt. II, ch. 17, subchptr. I, sec. 1705: Management of Health Care: Patient Enrollment System (www.law.cornell.edu/uscode/html/uscode38/usc_sec_38_00001705——000-.html).

14. Congressional Budget Office, *The Potential Cost of Meeting Demand for Veterans' Health Care* (CBO, March 2005), figure 3, p. 7.

15. Panangala, *Veterans' Medical Care Funding.*

16. Jonathan B. Perlin, under secretary of health, statement before the House Committee on Veterans' Affairs, Subcommittee on Health, 109th Cong., 2d sess., February 14, 2006.

17. DoD health funding is appropriated in different subaccounts that are combined in the annual reports and include total medical funding. Totals are provided for 1995, the first year of the TRICARE program, and for each year since 2000. Estimates of the total military health budget differ slightly depending on the methods used to identify health funding in nonhealth budget elements. The estimates used here are from a series of annual reports to Congress on TRICARE, which are available at http://tricare.osd.mil/ocfo/hpae/reports.cfm.

18. Congressional Budget Office, *Growth in Medical Spending by the Department of Defense* (2003).

19. Gary N. Nugent and others, "Value for Taxpayers' Dollars: What VA Care Would Cost at Medicare Prices," *Medical Care Research and Review* 61, no. 4 (2004): 495–508.

20. Steven Asch and others, "Comparison of Quality of Care for Patients in the Veterans Health Administration and Patients in a National Sample," *Annals of Internal Medicine* 141, no. 12 (December 2004): 938–45.

21. Eva A. Kerr and others, "Diabetes Care Quality in the Veterans Affairs Health Care System and Commercial Managed Care: The TRIAD Study," *Annals of Internal Medicine* 141, no. 4 (August 2004): 272–81.

22. Alfredo J. Selim and others, "Risk-Adjusted Mortality as an Indicator of Outcomes: Comparison of the Medicare Advantage Program with the Veterans' Health Administration," *Medical Care* 44, no. 4 (April 2006): 359–65.

23. Lucian L. Leape and Donald M. Berwick, "Five Years after *To Err Is Human:* What Have We Learned?" *Journal of the American Medical Association* 293, no. 19 (May 2005): 2384–390.

24. Mathew Goldberg, Ted Jaditz, and Viki Johnson, *Efficiency Analysis of Military Medical Treatment Facilities* (Alexandria, Va.: Center for Naval Analyses [CNA Corporation], October 2001).

25. U.S. Department of Defense, *The Economics of Sizing the Military Medical Establishment,* report of the comprehensive study of the military medical system (DoD, Office of Program Analysis and Evaluation, April 1994).

26. DoD, *Evaluation of the TRICARE Program: FY 2006 Report to Congress.*

27. Kaiser Family Foundation and Health Research and Educational Trust, *Employer Health Benefits: 2005 Annual Survey* (Washington: Kaiser Family Foundation and HRET, 2005).

28. Unlike TRICARE, the VHA does not cover dependents. Veterans with families who need to enroll in their employer plans to obtain dependent coverage will have less reason to use the VHA unless they have specialized health care needs.

29. TRICARE enrollment premium information can be found at "TRICARE Costs" (www.tricare.mil/tricarecost.cfm).

30. Geoffrey F. Joyce and others, "Employer Drug Benefit Plans and Spending on Prescription Drugs," *JAMA* 288, no. 14 (October 2002): 1733–739; Dana P. Goldman and others, "Pharmacy Benefits and the Use of Drugs by the Chronically Ill," *JAMA* 291, no. 19 (May 2004): 2344–350.

31. Roger Taylor and others, "Promoting Health Information Technology: Is There a Case for More-Aggressive Government Action?" *Health Affairs* 24, no. 5 (September-October 2005):1234–245.

32. VistA earned VHA the Innovations in American Government Award from the John F. Kennedy School of Government at Harvard University in July 2006.

33. Denise M. Hynes and others, "Informatics Resources to Support Health Care Quality Improvement in the Veterans Health Administration," *Journal of the American Medical Informatics Association* 11, no. 5 (June 2004): 344–50.

34. Aidan Hollis, "How Cheap Are Canada's Drugs Really?" *Journal of Pharmacy and Pharmaceutical Sciences* 7, no. 2 (2004): 215–16.

35. Ann E. Cook, "Strategies for Containing Drug Costs: Implications for a Medicare Benefit," *Health Care Financing Review* 20, no. 3 (1999): 29–37.

36. See Gail Wilensky's discussion in chapter 3 on Medicare and sustainable growth in health spending.

37. Susan D. Hosek and Garry Cecchine, *Reorganizing the Military Health System: Should There Be a Joint Command?* (Santa Monica, Calif.: RAND Corporation, 2001).

38. Luck and Peabody, "Improving the Public Sector: Can Reengineering Identify How to Boost Efficiency and Effectiveness at a VA Medical Center?"

6

Private Payer Roles in Moving to More Efficient Health Spending

PAUL B. GINSBURG

Developments in private insurance have direct and indirect effects on the federal budget and therefore strongly influence the degree to which measures to slow the growth of federal health spending can be successful. The private sector is even more important with respect to the broader goal of slowing the growth of total national health spending.

Direct and Indirect Effects

The direct interactions between private payers and the federal budget are mostly on the revenue side. The exclusion from taxation of employer contributions to employment-based health insurance is one of the largest tax expenditures in the federal budget. For fiscal year 2007, this expenditure is projected to total $146.8 billion. The Office of Management and Budget projects an increase of 45 percent between 2007 and 2011, substantially higher than the OMB's projection of increased total federal revenue of 26 percent over the same period.[1] Additional tax expenditures come from the deductibility of self-employed persons' purchase of health insurance coverage, employer or individual contributions to health savings accounts, and the medical expense deduction—also growing faster than federal revenues.

Direct subsidies for the purchase of private health insurance are becoming more important as well. In Medicare, beneficiaries can opt to obtain their coverage through a Medicare Advantage plan, which is administered by a private insurer, rather than through the traditional Medicare program. The recently implemented Medicare Part D program subsidizes the purchase of private coverage for prescription drugs. Some Medicaid programs, through federal waivers, subsidize the purchase of private coverage for categories of persons whose incomes are low but not low enough to qualify for regular Medicaid coverage. The federal government matches the cost of these subsidies.

Federal spending is also affected by the degree to which employment-based coverage is available to those who meet the qualifications for the Medicaid program. As employer-based coverage erodes over time, especially for relatively low-wage workers, more employed people (or at least their children) will be enrolling in Medicaid. To the degree that remaining employer-based coverage becomes less attractive to employees, both because contributions for coverage are higher and more patient cost sharing is required, more low-income workers with offers of coverage will nevertheless enroll in Medicaid.

A less direct and more speculative relationship concerns the degree to which higher costs and reduced access to private coverage will lead to political pressure for a major effort by the federal government to either expand public coverage or offer increased subsidies to private coverage. Although expanding health insurance coverage is not high on the federal policy agenda at this point, in a few years public demand could push the federal government to expand coverage along the lines of the recently enacted program in Massachusetts or actions of some other states.[2] The implication is that pressure for spending still more federal resources on health care may very well be on the horizon, spurred by increases in health spending that exceed people's ability to pay for care.

Less widely perceived are the indirect effects of developments in private insurance on federal spending for health care. Private insurance and the Medicare, Medicaid, and TRICARE programs all finance medical services from the same providers of services, including hospitals, physicians, freestanding outpatient facilities, and pharmaceutical manufacturers.[3] Although some providers, such as public hospitals and community health centers, treat low-income patients predominantly, most providers treat substantial numbers of patients covered by private insurance, Medicare, and Medicaid. Providers, for the most part, treat patients with different types of coverage the same way. If a hospital invests in expanding its facilities for high-end medical imaging, it is likely that care for both privately and publicly insured patients will include these services.

As a result of this common delivery system, it is likely that strong initiatives by one type of payer will influence the care for most patients, even those with distinct coverage. Although little research has been published, it is likely that the strong shift in enrollment among the privately insured to restrictive managed care products during the early 1990s had a spillover effect on Medicare and Medicaid. The authorization requirements of managed care plans for hospital admissions likely influenced physicians' admitting decisions for all of their patients. Hospitals may have put expansion plans on hold as a result of declining rates of admissions, at least for managed care patients. The need to offer greater discounts on rates to managed care plans may have made hospitals more cautious about spending for new technologies.

Moreover, overall trends in practice patterns in medical care affect all payers. If new medical technologies are covered by private payers, then a public payer will find it very difficult to not pay for them. The notion that public payers will only support a lower level of technology than is the norm in medical practice would violate long-held principles. As a practical matter, however, restriction of new technologies probably happens in Medicaid because providers are operating in difficult financial environments (many uninsured in addition to Medicaid patients).

This notion applies to public providers of care as well. The norms of care in private hospitals influence the expectations of the public for care in public facilities as well. For instance, Veterans Administration hospitals need to provide care comparable to that in private hospitals lest the Veterans Administration be accused of providing lower-quality care to our veterans.

Provider payment policies of private insurers may also influence what public insurers pay providers. Hospital administrators and insurers perceive that changes in payment rates by one major payer influence rates paid by other payers, although economists have puzzled over how this "cost shifting" can occur.[4] One reason is that private nonprofit hospitals often keep prices below those that would maximize revenues. They do this because of their nonprofit mission, the presence of community leaders on their boards, and concern about their image in the community. For-profit hospitals, however, which do not have these motivations, may be constrained by the rates charged by their more numerous nonprofit competitors.

On the one hand, if public payers reduce payment rates to hospitals and market conditions give hospitals enough power, then the hospital can offset the losses, at least in part, by raising rates to private payers. On the other hand, if hospitals do not have much power, as was the case in the mid-1990s when purchasers of insurance accepted narrow provider networks, then a reduction in rates by public payers might induce hospitals to reduce their costs instead of raising rates to private payers.[5]

Cost shifting can work both ways. Although most discussions have focused on the impact of Medicare and Medicaid payment policies on rates that private insurers pay, the relationship might go the other way. Public policymakers setting payment rates for Medicare or Medicaid are likely influenced by the financial status of hospitals. They are often called on to bail out foundering hospitals that are well regarded in their communities. The Medicare Payment Advisory Commission's annual tracking of trends in margins of hospitals is closely followed in Congress. Lower private rates could force hospitals to cut their costs to maintain their financial position. But if many hospitals experience deterioration in their financial position, it could influence public payers to be more generous. So if private payers are able to squeeze hospital rates, public payers might partly offset this by paying higher rates. Whether a cut in rates paid by private payers leads to higher or lower rates paid by the public programs depends upon whether hospital cost cutting, which would permit lower rates by public payers, or the policy response to deteriorating hospital financial positions predominates.

The relationship between private and public payment rates for physician services is distinct from the situation for hospital care. Public policymakers for the most part are not concerned with the financial status of physician practices, but they are concerned about physician acceptance of patients covered by public financing programs.[6] If private payment rates are high, this could either discourage or encourage acceptance of patients from public programs. Higher rates would make public patients relatively less attractive. But physicians often speak in terms of "target incomes," suggesting that higher rates for private patients could lead to greater ability to treat less lucrative patients with public coverage.

Provider reimbursement policies of private payers have been heavily influenced by Medicare policies and in turn have influenced Medicare policies. For physician payment, private payers have largely incorporated the Medicare structure of relative payment for different services. This has meant that changes in Medicare payment structures have the potential to have broader impacts on patterns of medical practice. But private payers' following the Medicare structure has probably also allowed the Medicare program to push further toward its goal of pegging its structure of payments based on its estimates of relative resource use because large discrepancies between public and private payment rates for specialties or categories of services are less likely to arise.

In recent years, the health care system has seen increasing examples of how innovations on the part of either private or public insurers influence the other. Private payers' experimentation with pay-for-performance (P4P) for physician services has increased public policymakers' interest in developing such a mechanism for the Medicare program. At about the same time, large employers and the Medicare program each experimented with the "centers of excellence" approach, which encouraged enrollees to use those providers with high quality of care ratings (with the private experience likely influencing the Medicare initiative). Unfortunately the approach has so far proved to have less potential than anticipated in both environments.[7] As another example, the experiences of private employers and insurers with disease management have influenced the Medicare program to pursue demonstrations of this approach. Indeed, expertise in disease management for employment-based coverage is easily transferable to

Medicare demonstrations, since vendors of disease management services as well as providers of care who have invested in this approach can be engaged in Medicare.

Private Payer Initiatives

Most private coverage is obtained through employment. The U.S. Census Bureau reports that 88 percent of private health insurance was obtained through employment in 2005.[8] In the absence of a public program for universal coverage, there are many strong reasons for linking private coverage to employment. Tax treatment of employment-based coverage confers a large subsidy to obtaining coverage through employment, with the subsidy generally greater for those with higher marginal income tax rates. Employers can obtain more favorable premiums than can individuals because employers are purchasing in bulk and because payroll deduction is a much lower-cost method of collecting regular payments from individuals than is monthly billing of enrollees. Employers' purchasing insurance for the majority of employees and their families permits them to vary employee contributions only by family status (single versus family coverage), meaning that older employees or those with chronic disease in their families are more likely to be able to afford coverage. Finally, employers provide valuable assistance to employees in navigating the purchase of a highly complex financial product.

The degree to which employers take major steps to contain the costs of the coverage they provide appears to be cyclical. During the early 1990s, when a deep recession led to low profits and slack labor markets, employers aggressively shifted their health benefits to managed care. In the late 1990s, with high profits and very tight labor markets, complaints about restrictions in managed care led to a shifting to less-restrictive versions. Authorization requirements for hospitalization or referral to a specialist or obtaining a major procedure were scaled back. Provider networks were expanded in response to demands for greater choice. It was or should have been clear that these steps would lead to higher costs. But health care premium trends were low at the time, and the urgent need was to address employee concerns.

Because of subsequently increasing premium trends and their recent experience with a recession, employers began to pay more attention to costs. Many stated that improved quality was the key to cost reduction, influenced perhaps by two landmark reports of the Institute of Medicine.[9] But employers continued to have concerns about antagonizing employees with aggressive management. Indeed, despite the enthusiasm of employers for the efforts of the Leapfrog Group, which promulgated quality standards for hospitals that employers should push for, many were unwilling to drop from their provider network those hospitals not meeting the standards.

Beginning in 2002, however, employers began to increase patient cost sharing in their health benefits plans. They increased deductibles, coinsurance, and co-payments but did not change the percentage of premiums contributed by employees. Their goal was to avoid discouraging enrollment while using shifts in financial responsibility to change behavior. Employers did not return to restrictive managed care, although authorization requirements were added to address specific problem areas, such as high-end imaging and specialty pharmaceuticals. This shift in cost sharing can be interpreted in two ways. One is that employers perceive the long-term outlook for labor markets to be relatively tight, especially for those with high skills, and shifting costs is more acceptable to those employees most difficult to retain than are administrative restrictions on care. The other is that society's attitude has shifted in favor of individuals making the key decisions in their health care as opposed to institutions, such as employers or insurers.

Patient Financial Incentives

The major thrust of cost containment strategies by employers today is to increase reliance on *patient financial incentives,* such as deductibles, coinsurance, and co-payments. Although good data to summarize the magnitude of change are not available, reports from Wall Street analysts that I have catalogued over time suggest that from 2001 to 2006 the actuarial value of private health insurance policies declined by more than 10 percent, with small employers experiencing larger declines in their policies.[10] Prescription drug benefits have perhaps changed the most. The norm has become a three-tiered structure with incentives to use generic drugs and those brand name drugs on a preferred list (brand name drugs not on the preferred list being the third tier). Some plans created a fourth tier for drugs that are deemed more elective than others (for example, drugs for erectile dysfunction) and for biologics, which are often so expensive that co-payments associated with the third tier are seen as having little impact on incentives. Over the course of this period, co-payments have increased, and coinsurance has been used increasingly instead of co-payments, with emphasis on increasing the magnitude of the incentives to favor the lower-cost tiers. Deductibles for both hospital and physician services have increased as well.

More attention has gone to *consumer-driven health plans,* which I define as plans with substantial patient financial incentives, a health savings account or health reimbursement account to pay medical bills, and consumer information tools on price and quality. Although enrollment has increased rapidly and surveys suggest that many large employers are offering or expect to offer such a plan, enrollment is still very small in relation to that of current employer-based coverage. America's Health Insurance Plans estimates that 3.2 million persons were enrolled in high-deductible health plans that were eligible for health savings accounts (HSAs) in January 2006.[11] In contrast, the Census Bureau estimates that 198.9 million had private insurance in 2005.[12] Much of the HSA coverage was in the market for individually purchased coverage, where the HSA is the only tax incentive that applies to those obtaining health insurance separately from employment. It is risky to extrapolate from a brief period of rapid growth of a new product.

Without doubt, increased patient financial incentives will reduce spending. The question is the magnitude of the impact. For example, if one compares standard actuarial assumptions with the 10 percent reduction in actuarial value noted above, the impact on spending might be around 2 percent—or 0.5 percent per year. Such an impact is not insignificant but is still relatively small in relation to the gap between spending trends and income trends, which historically has been 2.5 percentage points per year.[13] And there is a limit to the number of years that reductions in actuarial value can continue before insurance no longer provides substantial financial protection.

But the impact of increased financial incentives is likely greater than the standard assumptions would suggest because some of the response to the incentives is focused on choosing lower-priced providers. This was especially the case with prescription drugs, where cost sharing is structured to provide incentives to increase the use of generic drugs and those branded drugs that are in a preferred tier. Thus the response to higher drug co-payments in three-tiered structures would involve additional savings by shifting to less expensive drugs. However, benefit structures are not as oriented toward choosing hospital and physician services with lower prices, and information for consumers is very limited. This could change over time.

Nevertheless, a major question exists concerning the long-term impact of this core private-sector strategy. We know that health care spending in any year is concentrated in a minority of enrollees who have very large expenses. Ten percent of the population accounts for 69 percent of spending during the course of a year.[14] This means that a large proportion of spending will fall beyond the reach of patient financial incentives. These people will have exceeded their deductibles and limits on out-of-pocket spending. Should society continue in the direction of emphasizing patient financial incentives, benefit structures will need to evolve so that consumers can take more actions in the context of taking on a certain amount of financial risk.

These directions are starting to appear, although they are developing slowly. I believe that the direction offering greatest promise is to emphasize patient choice of provider. If a patient can be induced to choose a more efficient provider for an episode of care, then the incentive will have affected all of his or her spending for that episode—perhaps $100,000 worth of services rather than only the first $1,000.

A few years ago, insurers developed tiered hospital networks to create financial incentives to choose lower-cost hospitals. But hospital resistance (prominent hospitals threatened to leave networks unless they were placed in the preferred tier) and lack of employer interest have resulted in limited development. But *high-performance networks,* which focus on physicians in selected specialties, have had a much warmer reception by employers and are not as vulnerable to provider interference.

In a high-performance network, network physician practices in a specialty are sorted into two subnetworks. Patients are given financial incentives to favor those designated high performers. Typically, quality screens are used, then those practices passing the quality screens are ranked on the basis of costs per episode of care. These costs can include services beyond those provided by the physician, such as hospital costs, outpatient facility costs, and prescription drug costs. Direct savings are obtained when patients choose more efficient practices. If a significant share of the market adopts this tool, important indirect savings could be realized when those practices that are not high performers become more efficient to protect their patient volume.

This phenomenon is already happening in some areas. In Seattle, Aetna informed Virginia Mason Medical Center (VMMC), a large, integrated delivery system, that many of its specialties did not make the efficiency cut.[15] The two organizations began to work together to increase VMMC's efficiency so that it could remain in the preferred subnetwork, with Aetna providing analyses from its claims files and VMMC broadening its ongoing adoption of the Toyota Production System to focus on costs per episode.

High-performance networks are an example of a blending of consumerism and managed care. The managed care plan uses its data and analytical resources to assess the performance of providers and creates relatively simple financial incentives for consumers. But consumers can continue to access the providers who are not in the high-performance network and still benefit from negotiated payment rates and the lower cost sharing associated with using network providers.

The likely outcome—or at least the hoped-for outcome—of high-performance networks is that many providers will improve their efficiency and that public programs will benefit from the greater efficiency of providers who are treating their beneficiaries.

However, to the degree that the volume of services shifts toward the more efficient providers and that those providers do not expand their volume but instead respond by increasing the proportion of their patients with private insurance, spending by public programs could increase.

The federal government has an opportunity to spur development of this tool. A significant limiting factor for insurers is not having enough claims data for many practices to make reliable assessments of quality and efficiency. If the federal government provided access to Medicare claims data that identified the physician but not the beneficiary (other than a scrambled code to permit grouping of claims into episodes), insurers could use this tool more extensively. The federal government could also create a mechanism for private insurers to pool their own data for the purposes of having a larger sample with which each could make its own assessments of provider efficiency and quality.

Other potential strategies for implementing patient financial incentives would involve additional differentiation of cost sharing by type of service. The aim would be to avoid discouraging or burdening patients who use services that evidence suggests have substantial benefits and to place additional cost sharing for those services with small or uncertain benefits. Small steps are being taken in this direction. Some employers are reducing or eliminating cost sharing for services that are part of standard regimens for the management of chronic diseases—at least if the patient is participating in a disease management program. A well-known initiative is Pitney Bowes's reduction of drug co-payments to the rate for generic drugs for all drugs used in the treatment of diabetes, hypertension, and asthma. At the other end of the spectrum, some employers or insurers are setting higher coinsurance rates for certain procedures, such as bariatric surgery.

Employers' strategies that emphasize increasing financial incentives for patients will likely have impacts on federal programs. Medicaid enrollment will likely increase, especially for children, as parents see the virtue of substituting Medicaid for employment-based coverage. More extensive patient cost sharing could also increase political pressure to apply these changes to Medicare and Medicaid, given the contrasts between the benefit structure for Medicaid beneficiaries and that for those with somewhat higher incomes who have private coverage with extensive cost sharing. Hospitals are experiencing more bad debt from their patients who have more cost sharing. To the degree that policy on Medicare payment rates is based in part on the financial condition of hospitals, increased cost sharing in private insurance could lead to higher outlays for Medicare.

In theory, the Medicare and Medicaid programs could benefit from the development by private insurers of tools like high-performance networks and varying patient cost sharing by type of service. But they are not likely to transfer well. Congress has often discouraged the Centers for Medicare and Medicaid Services (CMS) from exercising the flexibility and judg-ment involved in initiatives like these, since some providers who are con-stituents perceive an entitlement to participate in these programs. In the case of Medicaid programs, low incomes of beneficiaries limit how exten-sively patient financial incentives can be used, although the current administration has been more open to such incentives, particularly for those beneficiaries with relatively high incomes. An important question concerning the Medicare program is the degree to which Medicare Advantage plans can incorporate some of these features without violating the rules on benefit structures.

If the use of patient financial incentives increases substantially, it could have some long-term impacts beyond direct responses by patients. For example, on the one hand, physicians would likely become more aware of affordability issues experienced by their patients and thus essentially increase their scope as agents for their patients, paying more attention to the patient costs for different drug alternatives or being less aggressive in ordering expensive diagnostic tests. On the other hand, if higher cost sharing leaves physicians less busy, they might prescribe their own ser-vices more readily.

Provider Reimbursement Methods

Private insurers have not been as innovative when it comes to provider reimbursement as has been the case in developing patient financial incen-tives. For the most part, insurers have adopted Medicare methods, screened billed charges for reasonableness, or negotiated discounts from charges. For example, with physician services, most private insurers use fee schedules based on the Medicare relative value scale. For small prac-tices, insurers' fee schedules are a percentage of Medicare rates, with the percentage varying widely by market. Fee schedules for larger practices tend to be negotiated but are also based on the Medicare structure. For inpatient care, diagnosis-related groups (DRGs) are not used extensively by private insurers. Payment tends to be either a discount from billed charges or a per diem payment. Like Medicare DRGs, per diem systems have a provision for additional payments for patients who use much greater amounts of services than the norm. Virtually all payment rates to hospitals are negotiated. Private insurers have slowly adopted prospective payment systems for other types of providers, as Medicare has developed them.

Interviews with provider relations executives at insurers revealed that few resources are devoted to innovating provider payment.[16] Many insurers believe that they do not have the clout to depart from either billed charges or Medicare methods, believing that providers would not agree to another structure of rates. But the fact that many insurers do follow Medicare methods means that Medicare reimbursement policies can more aggressively depart from established patterns of billed charges. It also means that when Medicare policies have a particular objective in mind, such as encouraging or discouraging types of services, their impact on the delivery system can be greater.

Incentives to Promote Higher Quality of Care

Increasing evidence that quality of care is not as high as it should be has spawned efforts to measure and report more indicators of quality and to incorporate quality into provider payment. For hospital care, Medicare has taken the lead in measurement and reporting through its voluntary hospital reporting standards. Hospitals now report on a series of measures specified by CMS, which are available to the public. Interviews with hospital officials have indicated that having these hospital quality measures publicly reported has motivated hospitals to improve quality.[17] Hospitals envision a future when private insurers use the information to steer enrollees to hospitals with higher quality scores.

For physicians, some private insurers are paying more when quality indicators are met. Pioneering work in pay-for-performance has been done in California by the Integrated Healthcare Association. Under the auspices of this voluntary organization, physician organizations and insurers collaboratively developed a uniform series of measures of quality on which each insurer would base its schedule of performance incentives. At this point, substantial payments are being made to practices that score higher.

A key challenge for private insurers has been coordinating the choice of measurements. Physicians understandably object to different sets of measures from each insurer. They also want a role in choosing the measures so that they have a degree of confidence in the standards on which payments will be made.

In the Boston area, P4P is used by each of the three major insurers without a need to coordinate on measurements of provider performance. This is because the insurers have limited their assessments of quality to information already available in standard claims data. Indeed, an important part of P4P in Boston is based on measures of cost, such as rates of imaging services ordered and the proportion of prescriptions that are for generic drugs. Boston insurers envision their system as not just a device to encourage better quality but also as something to replace the extensive use of capitation payments that had rapidly fallen out of favor.

The need for the coordination of measurements points to a significant potential role in this area for the Medicare program. Currently, CMS is conducting a number of demonstrations of P4P in Medicare. Congress has been debating whether to use P4P in the Medicare program and decided to pay physicians to report data on quality. It is likely that private insurers will coalesce around the specific reporting measures chosen by Medicare. Medicare's process of developing measures will certainly involve organized medicine, thereby making such measures more likely to be credible to practicing physicians. Indeed, the possibility that Congress might direct Medicare to pay on the basis of performance has spurred many specialty societies to develop measures relevant to their specialty that Medicare could adopt. With early versions of P4P focused mostly on primary care, specialists are strongly motivated to ensure that they also have opportunities for additional payments.

Should Medicare take the lead in P4P, followed by private payers, changes in physician incentives would be substantial. But the implications for spending are not clear. P4P in its early stages would likely include only bonuses for good performance and not penalties for poor performance. Changes in physician behavior in response to these incentives would likely improve quality, although how strong is the connection between process quality measures and outcomes is open to debate. But it is much more uncertain what the impact on spending would be. In addition to the P4P bonuses, some additional services that are paid separately would be performed more frequently. The unknown is whether some of the quality improvements would reduce the need for future services. Over time, it seems inevitable that a system with a series of bonuses but no penalties would erode the base payment rates—that is, payment rates, before performance incentives are paid, are likely to be increased less in the future in response to the cost of bonuses.

P4P could also significantly spur the adoption of information technology by physicians, if Medicare required or strongly encouraged physician reporting of quality measures in electronic form. The indirect result could be savings in other areas, such as reduction in the duplication of tests or fewer medical errors. If large practices, because of their infrastructure, tended to capture much higher rates of P4P bonuses than did small practices, this could accelerate the ongoing movement of physicians from small to large practices, a change that could have positive implications for costs and quality.

Disease Management and Wellness

In recent years, disease management (DM) programs have become a more significant part of the landscape in private insurance. Disease management programs tend to be designed to support physicians with complementary resources, such as patient monitoring and education. Their use has long been driven by employer or insurer demands for evidence that it pays for itself in reduced medical spending. The evolution of DM has involved focusing on patients with a higher likelihood of benefiting, for example, instead of all diabetics, focus on those with more severe disease. It has also involved choosing diseases on the basis of disease patterns in an employer's workforce. The benefits to employers and insurers of disease management are limited by turnover. Returns to these investments are lost when an employee changes jobs or health plans. Some important benefits of disease management are probably ignored because most employers are unable to measure benefits of reduced disability and absenteeism and higher productivity while on the job.

Little research on the effectiveness of DM has appeared in peer-reviewed journals. This could reflect the rapidly changing mechanisms used or a lack of financial support for careful objective studies. It appears that DM companies have been able to present enough evidence to employers and insurers to justify the continuation and expansion of disease management. However, the returns do not appear to be very large. DM might be effective enough to more than pay for itself, but it is unlikely to be a potential solution to the broader health spending issue.

Medicare has been conducting extensive demonstrations in DM for a number of years. There are factors that suggest that the tool could either be more or less effective in Medicare than in employer-based coverage. The low rate of turnover in the Medicare population is clearly a plus, since more of the gains from the investment can be captured by the program. The fact that an elderly population has a higher incidence of chronic disease presents a substantial opportunity for DM to have an effect. However, the gains that employers can realize from reduced absenteeism and disability do not apply here.

Employers have invested in DM on the basis of very limited information on its effectiveness. This could be a problem for Medicare, where officials do not have the opportunities that private-sector benefits managers have to pursue initiatives with only limited research evidence to support it. This helps explain why CMS has invested a lot in demonstrations of DM—it needs successful demonstrations before it can contemplate much broader application.

Further development by private payers of DM tools will have benefits for the Medicare program. The more effective the tools are, the more likely that the Medicare program will be able to employ them. Transferring the technology should not be a problem, since either DM vendors or private insurers who conduct DM with their own staffs can be hired as contractors in Medicare.

Recently, employers have become more interested in promoting wellness in their workforces. However, the field appears to be highly fragmented; it has not coalesced around a small number of tools that are seen as particularly effective. One tool that has recently garnered interest has been the health assessment. Some employers have pushed employees to take the assessment, using either bonuses or penalties. In King County, Washington, the local government has gotten a lot of attention for not only using incentives to encourage employees' taking the assessment, but also for attaching rewards for following the advice given in the assessment. The field of wellness seems to be at a much earlier stage than is DM and is probably less likely to be applied to Medicare in the near future.

Conclusion

The outlook for federal spending on health care is substantially inter-twined with developments in private health insurance. Beneficiaries of federal programs and enrollees in private coverage get their care from a common health care delivery system. Federal programs cannot succeed by pushing the delivery system in directions that are at odds with directions pursued by private payers. There are important opportunities for tools used in the public or private sector to contain spending to make similar efforts more effective in the other sector. Public and private insurers today are very familiar with the tools of their counterparts and more open to adapting them than has been the case in the past.

At this point in time, greater use of patient financial incentives, coupled with providing patients with information on provider price and quality, is the key strategy of private payers. The public sector is not pursuing such a strategy, and it does not have a clear strategy of its own, except for the current administration's strategy of increasing the use of private insurance in public programs. However, a number of public-sector activities have the potential to facilitate private-sector strategies and possibly have some favorable direct effects on the private-sector delivery system. These activities include revamping provider reimbursement to reduce inadvertent incentives to expand certain services and promoting measurement and reporting of provider quality.

Notes

1. Office of Management and Budget, *Analytical Perspectives: Budget of the United States Government, Fiscal Year 2007* (Government Printing Office, 2006). These estimates refer to foregone federal income tax revenue only and do not include foregone revenue from federal payroll taxes or state income taxes.

2. In 2006 Massachusetts enacted a series of policies designed to substantially reduce the proportion of the population who are uninsured. The policies included an expansion of public coverage for low-income persons, subsidies to purchase private insurance, fees to be assessed on employers who do not provide coverage,

a mechanism to increase the efficiency of the insurance market for small groups and individual purchasers, and a mandate on individuals to have coverage.

3. The TRICARE program provides private insurance for military dependents and retirees.

4. Paul B. Ginsburg, "Can Hospitals and Physicians Shift the Effects of Cuts in Medicare Reimbursement to Private Payers?" *Health Affairs* web exclusive, October 8, 2003: W3-472–W3-479.

5. A network is a listing of medical providers who have a contract with the insurer to provide services to enrollees at a negotiated price. The terms "broad" or "narrow" refer to extensive or limited degrees of provider choice.

6. Policymakers are becoming concerned about how declines in physician income in primary care have resulted in fewer physicians entering into those specialties. Similar concerns in the mid-1980s led to reform of physician payment in Medicare, which was enacted in 1989.

7. Private employers found employee interest in centers of excellence to be much lower than anticipated. Medicare was not able to translate its successful demonstration of the approach for coronary artery bypass graft surgery (CABG) into demonstrations for other procedures, perhaps because the ease in measurement of provider quality and the substantial variation in provider quality are not found in many other important procedures. When variation in quality is small, less is gained by pushing consumers to use the better providers.

8. Census Bureau, Current Population Survey, 2006 Annual Social and Economic Supplement, Table HI01, "Health Insurance Coverage Status and Type of Coverage by Selected Characteristics: 2005, All Races," http://pubdb3.census.gov/macro/032006/health/h01_001.htm.

9. Linda T. Kohn, Janet M. Corrigan, and Molla S. Donaldson, eds., *To Err is Human: Building a Safer Health System* (Washington: Committee on Quality of Health Care in America, Institute of Medicine, National Academy Press, 2000); Committee on Quality of Health Care in America, *Crossing The Quality Chasm: A New Health System For The 21st Century* (Washington: Institute of Medicine, National Academy Press, 2001).

10. Although some employer surveys do include detailed questions on the benefit structures of health plans and actuaries have models to summarize this information into an actuarial value, the dynamism of benefit structures leads this approach to underestimate changes. When a new type of cost sharing is introduced, its impact will not be measured during the period from its introduction until it is recognized as pervasive enough to include in survey questionnaires.

11. America's Health Insurance Plans, "January 2006 Census Shows 3.2 Million People Covered by HSA Plans" (Washington: AHIP, Center for Policy and Research, 2006).

12. Census Bureau, Current Population Survey, 2006 Annual Social and Economic Supplement, Table HI01.

13. Calculations by the author from National Health Accounts data published by the Centers for Medicare and Medicaid Services.

14. Marc L. Berk and Alan C. Monheit, "The Concentration of Health Care Expenditures, Revisited," *Health Affairs* 20, no. 2 (March-April 2001): 9–18.

15. The Center for Studying Health System Change is studying this experience with support from the California HealthCare Foundation. The discussion here is limited to information that has been covered in public presentations by officials from Aetna or the Virginia Mason Medical Center.

16. Paul B. Ginsburg and Joy M. Grossman, "When the Price Isn't Right: How Inadvertent Payment Incentives Drive Medical Care," *Health Affairs* web exclusive, August 9, 2005: W5-376–W5-384.

17. Hoangmai H. Pham, Jennifer Coughlan, Ann S. O'Malley, "The Impact of Quality-Reporting Programs on Hospital Operations," *Health Affairs* 25, no. 5 (September-October 2006): 1412–422.

7

Cost Containment and the Politics of Health Care Reform

JUDITH FEDER AND DONALD W. MORAN

A s the diverse array of viewpoints expressed in the foregoing chapters makes clear, "health care reform"—even with the more specific goal of cost containment—means different things to different people. As a political catchphrase, health care reform garners nearly universal support, since individual observers view the issue through the lens of their own policy preferences. In virtually every federal election since the 1960s, the "health care issue" has polled near the top of the public's concerns.

Despite this fact, precious little that most serious analysts would consider reform actually seems to get done. While our political system has shown a willingness to busy itself about the margins of programs of public-sector health care financing, efforts to reform the broader health care financing and delivery systems have proven largely ineffectual despite nearly universal support, at least in the abstract, for such efforts.

To understand why this happens, we trace what we believe are the major impediments to large-scale reform through the last two decades of national political experience and then offer our conclusions, in light of this experience, about what needs to happen to make successful reform occur.

The Legacy of the Clinton Reform Plan

Two vivid images stand out from the early years of the Clinton administration. The first is "It's the economy, stupid," the mantra of the 1992 Clinton presidential campaign. Slowing the growth of health care costs was central to Clinton's strategy for restoring the nation's economic health. Second is President Bill Clinton lifting his pen before a joint session of Congress, emphatically asserting his commitment to veto any health insurance legislation that failed to provide universal coverage. Costs and coverage were integrally intertwined in the Clinton administration's health reform. This is a political as well as a policy relationship, driven by the reality of health care financing—that unless there is a willingness to spend more money, it is not possible to cover the uninsured without placing restrictions on the already insured. This reality stalled movement toward national health insurance after Medicare's enactment, simultaneously motivated and doomed the Clinton health reform plan, and not only impedes efforts to expand coverage today but actually contributes to its demise. This section reviews the emergence of the cost-coverage connection in the 1960s, illustrates its role in both motivating and destroying the Clinton plan, and examines the political stalemate it creates today.[1]

The Buildup to Reform

The social insurance activists who designed Medicare saw its 1965 enactment as a step—hopefully a large one—toward national health insurance, modeled on Social Security. Instead, Medicare's (and with it Medicaid's) enactment established an institutional and fiscal path that impedes, rather than facilitates, universal coverage.

As institutions, Medicare and Medicaid are the public side of a public-private partnership that insures 85 percent of Americans. This insured population powerfully resists changes to the existing structure, which systematically excludes the low- and modest-income uninsured. The private side of that partnership emerged in the 1940s and 1950s, as multiple forces combined to produce employer-sponsored health insurance:

—the labor movement's shift from national politics to collective bargaining as the way to gain health insurance;

—business interests' preferences for fringe benefits over government-run (or labor-organized) health insurance;

—insurance industry capacity for and interest in providing those benefits; and

—administrative action, backed by legislation establishing tax preferences—most important, the exclusion of employer-paid premiums from employee taxable income—that subsidized employer-sponsored health insurance.[2]

Establishment of employer-sponsored health insurance, in turn, created a case for adding public health insurance for the nonworking population. Beginning in the 1950s, national health insurance advocates shifted their attention away from the general population and toward the elderly—a politically attractive group "deserving" of public protection and unlikely to be reached by work-based or other private health insurance. The political compromise that established Medicare as universal social insurance for the elderly also established Medicaid as means-tested health insurance for certain population subgroups—specifically, low-income persons who received cash assistance because of age, blindness, disability, or (in the case of children living with single mothers) "dependency" status.[3] The result was creation of a public health insurance system targeted to people not expected to work and built around the private, albeit tax-subsidized, insurance system for workers and their families.

Employer-sponsored health insurance expanded dramatically to cover a growing share of workers and their families through the 1970s. But then growth stopped. The numbers—and the proportion—of working-aged Americans without health insurance coverage have grown steadily from that time forward.[4] Even when the economy is booming, employer-sponsored insurance fails to reach millions of low- and modest-wage workers in both large and small firms.

The public health insurance system also grew in the second half of the twentieth century. Very shortly after its enactment, Medicare extended coverage to disabled beneficiaries of Social Security and people with end-stage renal disease.[5] And although its coverage was immediately narrowed, Medicaid has grown enormously and is now the nation's largest insurance program, covering more than 50 million people. In the 1980s and early 1990s, growth came primarily through the extension of eligibility standards beyond cash assistance standards for children and pregnant women. More modestly and more recently, growth came through the 1996 enactment of the State Children's Health Insurance Program. Medicaid covers the low-income aged and disabled persons, but the bulk of its enrollees are children and, to a much lesser extent, their mothers. For the most part Medicaid excludes low-income workers.[6]

Overall, employer-sponsored insurance and the public programs designed primarily for people outside the workforce—Medicare and Medicaid—cover about 85 percent of our population. However, by their explicit structures they exclude people who work but who are not offered health insurance through their jobs and who, primarily because they work, remain outside the categories covered by public programs.

Why is that a barrier to coverage expansions? Although it is true that any person can fall out of employer-sponsored coverage—by, for example, losing a job or getting divorced—the vast majority of Americans can count on receiving health insurance through the workplace. The primary political and policy problems are that it is almost impossible to insure the "have-nots" without in some way disrupting the status quo of the "haves."

The fiscal path established with the nation's public-private insurance system is at the core of that disruption. This system has fueled an escalation of health care costs that not only strains the nation's economic and political capacity to guarantee universal coverage, but it also threatens to unravel the coverage Americans already have. The fault lies not with the public programs—rather, the problem is intrinsic to insurance. Protecting people against the costs of illness (the fundamental purpose of insurance) removes sensitivity to price as a constraint on care. Unless insurers, public or private, find ways to constrain what they pay, costs are destined to rise—whether through support for technology that demonstrably improves the public's health or through inefficiency and waste in the system.

Despite payment reforms that have made Medicare, if anything, more effective than the private sector in containing costs, the "crisis" of rising health care costs first declared in 1972 by President Richard Nixon persists today.[7] Clearly, the "cost crisis" comes from service to those who have health insurance, not from those who do not. But rising costs create an enormous barrier to coverage expansion. First, rising health care costs contribute to growth in the number of uninsured, as premiums become less affordable to employers and individual purchasers.[8] Second, rising costs raise the political, as well as the economic, costs of political action to expand coverage. The full cost of employer-sponsored coverage of a typical family is now more than $11,000 per year.[9] If comparable insurance were available to individuals outside employment, it would absorb more than 20 percent of income for the bulk of the uninsured. Virtually every health insurance expansion proposal, regardless of its form, recognizes that the cost of health insurance is too high to expect the uninsured to purchase it without subsidies. Higher health care costs mean more expensive subsidies, which increase the resources that must inevitably be shifted from those who have health insurance to those who are without.

This redistribution has always been a hard sell, and it gets harder the more it costs and the more the better-off insured have to pay for their own health insurance and health care. Politically, the uninsured are held hostage to the unwillingness of the insured to control their health care costs. The Clinton experience is a good example of this situation.

The Clinton Coverage Strategy

Reluctance to disrupt Americans who have health insurance, whether through redistribution or changes in health care that universal coverage might bring, has inhibited most politicians from directly taking on displacement. The Clinton health reform proposal focused at least as much on those who had health insurance as on those who lacked it and assiduously tried to avoid private-to-public coverage shifts.

Cost containment was the motivator and the linchpin of this strategy. Clinton saw slowing the growth of health care costs as essential to achieving the critical goals of balancing the federal budget and growing the economy. Universal coverage became part of that strategy—necessary to ensure that slower spending came not from reductions in coverage, or shifts in costs from one payer to another, but instead from greater efficiency in purchasing care. The fundamental challenge in achieving this strategy was finding a way to cover everyone, including the then 37 million uninsured, while also slowing health care spending in general and avoiding increases in public spending in particular.

The Clinton health plan built universal coverage by securing and extending existing employer-sponsored insurance through an employer mandate. All employers would have been required to provide coverage for their workers at benefit levels that matched those held by the well-insured. This mandate aimed to appeal to the currently covered in two ways. First, the requirement that employers provide comprehensive coverage secured the health benefits that workers were afraid of losing in a weak economy. Second, because most of the uninsured were working, the mandate meant that employers and employees would bear the immediate responsibility for paying for the expansion without having to impose new taxes on the already-insured.[10]

The Clinton proposal also contained an approach for financing subsidies for lower-income families without imposing new taxes.[11] Public funds to finance these subsidies—and others included in the proposal, such as those to finance coverage for the minority of uninsured persons outside the workforce—would have been generated through aggressive cost containment, which would produce savings in federal health programs that could be reinvested. It was estimated that slower growth in health costs would reduce projected federal spending (which was most important for Medicaid) and also would reduce federal revenue losses or "tax expenditures" for employer-sponsored health insurance.[12] Lower-than-projected public expenditures and higher-than-expected tax revenues made room in the federal budget to finance the new subsidies that were essential to the success of the Clinton plan.

To gain sufficient room in the federal budget, growth in health care costs had to be held to levels of general inflation—a level never previously achieved. The Clinton administration advocated "managed competition" for this purpose. Specifically, the proposal sought to guarantee everyone 80 percent of the average cost of a choice of health plans, all of which offered a guaranteed scope of benefits and uniform cost sharing. These competing plans would be made available to consumers through newly structured and highly regulated insurance markets, labeled "alliances." Consumers—either directly or in very large firms through their place of employment—would shop for, and financially benefit from, selecting a lower-cost plan. The theory was that insurers would compete for consumers by keeping their costs down. Prohibited from competing on benefit levels or by avoiding high-risk enrollees, plans would be forced to compete by securing efficient delivery of quality care.

Under the congressional budget rules then in place, the Congressional Budget Office (CBO) was responsible for determining whether the Clinton proposal provided sufficient financing to cover its costs. CBO did not share the high expectations of the Clinton administration and other proposal proponents for cost containment through managed competition. Avoiding the need for new revenues and satisfying CBO required including what the proposal designers saw as a "backup" mechanism: caps on the rate of growth in insurance premiums, enforced through reductions (as necessary) in provider payments.

Mandatory contributions from employers and individuals, accompanied by aggressive cost containment to produce federal budget savings, enabled the Clinton administration to claim that it guaranteed health insurance to all Americans at no new federal cost and that over the next 10 years it would actually lead to lower health care costs for the nation than would have occurred in its absence.[13]

The administration believed this strategy would not only create a healthier nation; it would overcome the long-standing political obstacles to reform posed by resistance to redistribution from and disruption of the already-insured. But the Clinton strategy was no more successful than previous national health insurance efforts at avoiding controversy about disruption and redistribution. Interest groups for whom cost containment meant revenue loss joined forces with ideological opponents of the Clinton reform to support a massive lobbying campaign against its enactment. That campaign successfully reframed the health reform debate, shifting attention from the benefits to the risks of reform, making it safer for politicians to support the status quo.

Rather than being welcomed as simplifying and securing private coverage, the Clinton proposal's new insurance markets were attacked as big government interference with employer-sponsored insurance. Rather than being applauded for reducing the growth of health care costs, the Clinton proposal's cost containment was criticized as rationing care. Rather than making everyone a winner, as its designers intended, the plan was characterized as making losers of all who already had insurance, in terms of access to quality care, in no small part because their health benefits would be subject to aggregate, alliance-wide standards and the cost of their coverage subject to aggregate controls. At the end of the Clinton health reform debate, polls indicated that only about one in five Americans believed reform would make them better-off—in general and with respect to quality of care. A far larger proportion—more than one in three—believed they would be worse-off from enactment of the proposed health reform.[14]

It was undoubtedly these concerns that led the public to resonate with advertisements run by the Health Insurance Association of America featuring an all-American couple named Harry and Louise, who memorably lamented, "There's got to be a better way."[15] But, holding the specifics of the Clinton plan aside, the truth is there simply is no way to design a universal coverage policy that can cover the uninsured without affecting the already-insured; and no way to achieve political success if the already-insured perceive that they would be worse-off as a result. Even if "new" revenues are identified in an attempt to finance new coverage without diminution of current coverage, all of the presently-insured would still be materially affected by whatever cost containment strategy was established to hold the total costs within the expanded resource envelope thus created. The experience of the Clinton era reinforces the conclusion that it is structurally impossible to expand coverage in a way that all actors in the health care system would consider "free." That being the case, relief for the 15 percent of the population without coverage will only arrive if the bargain fashioned to achieve that coverage looks reasonable to the 85 percent of the population who are satisfied with, but concerned about the security and continuation of, their existing health care coverage

Political Realities Today

Coming forward from the experiences of the Clinton era, it is apparent that wherever U.S. health care policy is headed it will make its way forward in an increasingly polarized environment.

Since at least the Bush-Gore election finale in 2000, U.S. politics has become acutely polarized, both from the perspective of traditional inter-party warfare and a more recent factionalism that pits opposing ideological orthodoxies against each other on virtually every front.[16] Issues arising in health care are, not surprisingly, as susceptible to factionaliza-tion as any other issue of public discourse. Yet health care interacts with American political discourse in some distinctive ways.

First, several of the hot button social issues that mobilize activism across the ideological divide lie inextricably within the health care realm. The legality of abortion services has dominated debate over reproductive health issues since the early 1970s. More recently, the controversy over the ethics and federal funding of stem cell research has opened yet another factional front within health research policy.

Second, the growing fiscal importance of public and private spending on health care services (well documented in preceding chapters) has come to dominate political agendas at the state and federal levels. As more and more of what government does involves setting health care policy, it is natural that both partisan and ideological battles spill over into this arena.

Third, the increasingly perceived disappearance of the center in politics has particularly strong effects in health care policy.[17] Given the size and complexity of the health care system, a substantial amount of year-to-year legislative and regulatory action is needed simply to keep the existing pro-grammatic framework running smoothly. For most of the last forty years, since the enactment of Medicare and Medicaid, there has been a sufficient core of lawmakers in both parties who—regardless of where they stood on the major thematic battles of their times—were willing to work together to keep the trains running smoothly.

Increasingly, however, partisans of various factions seek to use every available vehicle to advance hot button priorities from their ends of the polar divide. This tendency has become increasingly evident since enact-ment of legislation to implement the new Medicare prescription drug benefit.

The Politics of the Medicare Modernization Act

When Medicare was first enacted in 1965, no thought was given to pro-viding coverage for prescription drugs because, frankly, there was not much to cover. The limited number of prescription drugs available at that time—notably antibiotics and vaccines—were commonly injected in physi-cian offices rather than sold through pharmacies. Hence, the prevailing mode of Medicare coverage for prescription drugs dealt only with drugs administered "incident to" physician services.

By the mid-1980s, however, the widening availability of clinically effective oral medications changed public perceptions of the adequacy of the Medicare drug benefit. The growth of explicit outpatient prescription drug coverage through managed care organizations, in particular, created pressure to provide all Medicare beneficiaries with a comparable benefit.

The first effort to do so is widely acknowledged as one of the great political reversals in the history of health policy.[18] The Medicare Catastrophic Coverage Act (MCAA) of 1988 conferred new Medicare benefits, in the form of increased protection against excessive out-of-pocket costs for acute medical-surgical services, as well as first-time-ever coverage for outpatient prescription drug subscriptions filled in pharmacies.[19] In the "pay as you go" spirit of the late Reagan era, the incremental cost of these benefits was to be financed by new income-related premiums administered by mandatory deductions from the beneficiaries' Social Security benefits. Since many elderly beneficiaries already had some form of coverage for cost sharing and drug coverage that at least partially duplicated the new MCCA benefits, these "Social Security taxes" triggered a revolt against the program that caused nervous lawmakers to repeal the entire statute before implementation.

While analysts drew different conclusions from this sequence of events, one notable subplot was the role of the pharmaceutical industry in shaping the final product.[20] Concerned about the prospect of drug price controls, the Pharmaceutical Research and Manufacturers of America (PhRMA) actively campaigned against the bill until all references to price-related policy adjustments were stripped from the final legislation. Hence policymakers reached the conclusion that when it came to outpatient prescription drug benefits, beneficiaries would refuse to pay for coverage and manufacturers were inalterably opposed to any version that provided an explicit cost containment mechanism—which most fiscal analysts perceived to be a *sine qua non* of an effective program.

This lingering perception dominated health policymaking in Washington for the next decade. Despite rapidly rising drug use by the elderly—and rapidly rising drug costs—drug coverage under the regular Medicare benefit was broadly understood to be politically unworkable.[21]

This perception changed in 1999 with the Medicare reform program generated, but not formally adopted, by a National Bipartisan Commission on the Future of Medicare.[22] The central controversy revolved around the report's proposal of a historic quid pro quo: a prescription drug benefit would be added to Medicare, but the basic Medicare benefit would be converted from a defined benefit to a defined contribution model, under which Medicare would offer each beneficiary a fixed level of premium support that the beneficiary could use to select among benefit options requiring greater or lesser amounts of supplemental premium payments.[23] This recommendation, which was understood by all parties to represent a marked departure from the social insurance character of the Medicare program as originally enacted, became the fault line for the ensuing debate.[24]

For conservatives, the drug benefit recommended by the Breaux-Thomas model was understood as the reluctant price to be paid for conversion of Medicare to what was perceived to be a more stable fiscal model.[25] Social insurance activists, by contrast, saw an opportunity to press for modernization of the Medicare program via a drug benefit—while at the same time strongly opposing any effort to modify the defined benefit structure of the program. Since both sides of the divide saw merit in pushing toward a drug benefit, the debate shifted from the pro quo of the benefits controversy to the quid of a free-standing prescription drug program.

This tilt in direction was—at least passively—enabled by the pharmaceutical industry, which endorsed the notion of a Medicare drug benefit *in the context of market-based reforms of the Medicare program*.[26] At the time, this characterization was perceived as an endorsement by PhRMA of the premium support model embodied in the Breaux-Thomas recommendations. As will be seen, however, PhRMA's position ultimately proved more flexible than the pure quid pro quo position embraced by conservatives.

In the ensuing four years, the health policy debate in Washington was anchored around the advance of legislation implementing a drug benefit. Quite quickly, the debate over a free-standing benefit transformed into a stylized argument over high-level design principles. Republicans, who were nominally at the wheel because of their control of both the White

House and the House of Representatives, promoted designs based on choices among options in a pluralistic private market.[27] Democrats differed on how pluralistic the model might be but coalesced around the notion that a centralized federal plan should be available as an option and that it should have the authority to negotiate drug prices with manufacturers. PhRMA, while not actively supporting any particular approach, did not object to discussions of a free-standing option as long as its codicil regarding private-market administration of that benefit was honored.

When the debate began, it arose in the context of unprecedented budget harmony at the federal level; in 1999 budget surpluses totaling $5.6 trillion were forecast for the ten-year budget horizon. As debate wore on, however, the projected surplus proved ephemeral, and conservatives became increasingly concerned about the rising cost estimates for the program. Hence when the House passed its version of the plan in 2003, House leaders added language providing for a phase-in of a Breaux–Thomas–style model of premium support beginning toward the end of the decade. While the quid pro quo view of the drug benefit had largely disappeared from the general policy landscape, it was alive and well in the House of Representatives.

That view in the Senate, however, was "deader than a doornail." A Senate bill could not have been fashioned without active support from Democratic leaders, who were not buying the notion that the debate was about anything other than a free-standing drug benefit for Medicare.[28]

It is not surprising, when these competing visions clashed in conference, that the dissonance was substantial. Ultimately, eleven Democratic senators were convinced to sign on when any semblance of the House quid pro quo was thrown over the side.[29] While this neatly solved the problem in the Senate, it created a firestorm in the conservative wing of the House, who saw their trump card—acquiescence in a drug benefit—about to be cashed for no net gain.

The resulting saga of the House passage of the conference report will long be studied as a natural experiment in tactical legislative engineering. Since the Senate had already passed the product, and was unlikely to pass another, House leaders found themselves in a "one suit squeeze," in which they had to put together 218 votes for passage without the ability to add inducements to the bill to cushion the agony for conservatives of voting for what they suspected to be a fiscal disaster waiting to happen. After keeping the final vote open for hours, House leaders ultimately found enough Democrats to join the remaining Republicans and pass the conference agreement. The fallout from the experience just described, occurring as it did in an environment that was already politically and ideologically polarized, sets the stage for substantial challenges going forward.

First, with respect to the drug benefit itself, the normal political posture that might be expected upon passage of a major new entitlement was inverted. In the emerging political order, Democrats apparently see political advantage in heaping scorn upon an entitlement program that Republicans amazedly find themselves championing as their major domestic policy accomplishment. It seems likely that Democratic efforts to amend the programmatic status quo that Republicans now find themselves reflexively defending will materially affect both legislative and regulatory tactics in health policy for many years to come.

Second, it means that as leaders in both parties look forward to the impending fiscal crisis in both public and private health care finance, it is not easy to visualize how to grow a political center large enough to take concerted action to restore fiscal sanity before the financial divide between promises and resources proves unbridgeable. Neither political party has a motive, in the current environment, to offer an olive branch on these issues to the other side. Thus the situation awaits individual leaders, in both parties, who can figure out how to frame the debate in a way that permits them to draw enough of their colleagues across present battle lines to form a working coalition to make fundamental changes in the fiscal terms of trade in health care.

Looking Forward

When these leaders come forward, what must their agenda be?

Based on our reading of the experience described above, we believe that progress on all fronts will be stymied until a framework can be created—as suggested in the preceding chapters—in which the health care system can get serious about cost containment.

We use this phrase with some trepidation, since admonitions to "get serious about cost containment" have been a staple in the health policy debate since at least the early 1970s. In such discourse, cost containment is invoked as if it were some monolithic strategy that would be uniformly efficacious in restraining the growth of health care costs, if only Congress were virtuous enough to invoke it. Yet cost containment is no more a strategy than is good government. As chapter 2 in this volume emphasizes, getting serious about cost containment means that the American political system must disavow the notion that such a magic bullet exists.

Costs in the American health care system are determined by hundreds of thousands—if not millions—of decisions made by individual Americans every day. Costs go up when a pharmaceutical manufacturer signs a contract to conduct a clinical trial of a promising but uncertain chemical compound. Costs go up when a hospital administrator decides to order a new 64-slice CT machine to replace an older piece of equipment that still performs to its original specifications. Costs go up and down when people in the system are hired, fired, or transferred to new assignments. And costs throughout the system ride heavily on the myriad decisions made each day to seek or not to seek care of various types.

To be serious about cost containment, it will be necessary to admit that containing costs will require affecting the decisions that individual Americans make every day in all the settings in which they make them. If this country wants a system that is more economical, lots of people will have to economize; perhaps everyone will. While we have demonstrated our capacity, as a society, to support devoting a growing level of real resources to the system each year, "everything someone can think of for anybody who asks" is neither desirable nor sustainable. Getting serious about cost containment will require policymakers to develop the evidence and the policy process that will allow the system to rationally and acceptably say no.

Getting to No

As we contemplate the prospect of whether the American political system can consciously accommodate economizing in health care, it is important to observe that, in the normal course of political business as usual, as the numbers of uninsured and underinsured continue to rise in the absence of policies designed to make broad-based insurance affordable, more and more Americans will face stark incentives to economize on health care

COST CONTAINMENT AND HEALTH CARE REFORM

each year. We will not have to advocate explicit rationing to keep the costs of treating the uninsured in check. Americans will do the rationing themselves, occasionally in ways that we might consider suboptimal from the perspective of costs to society as a whole. Increasingly, those who seek employment at establishments that do not offer insurance, together with those employed at establishments that embrace catastrophic-only insurance designs, will be in the free market for health care products and services. In that market, they will trade off health care services they would have previously consumed in a regime of insurance for other necessities and pleasures of life. They will, in truth, be serious about cost containment in ways that fully insured Americans hope that they will never have to adopt.

Unless those who design the nation's public and private health insurance systems get serious about cost containment, the drift toward this de facto "uninsured free market" cost containment model is likely to accelerate. Getting serious means developing strategies that go beyond a focus on the price of services to a focus on the value of services.

The private insurance sector has a mixed history in terms of seriousness about cost containment. After the sharp insurance premium run-up in the late 1980s, the private sector embraced managed care, which in theory attempted to steer patients to preferred providers and to actively control access to expensive technologies via discretionary, patient-by-patient decisionmaking. Although this strategy temporarily contained costs, concern that insurers cared more about managing costs than managing care—thereby putting patients at risk—produced a substantial political backlash against these models. Throughout the present decade, employers have responded by relaxing efforts to control premium costs, and instead they are decreasing what they would otherwise have provided to employees as compensation, such as wage growth or other benefits. The growth in employment at establishments that do not offer insurance, however, is a sign that this strategy too has its limits.[30]

In public insurance systems, serious cost containment has not been the dominant mode of operation. Public programs, notably Medicare, have shown a marked tendency to lower payment rates to providers, rather than attempting to steer decisionmaking by physicians and their patients toward more economical outcomes. The effectiveness of this strategy is limited by its perverse result of inducing providers to offset the income loss by increasing unit volumes of services ordered.

Serious Cost Containment in Insurance Systems

There are three types of control handles that could be used in public and private insurance systems to implement more serious efforts to promote cost-conscious decisionmaking.

First, insurance programs can manage cost exposure by managing coverage policy. Rather than routinely covering each new medical technology, insurers could tie coverage of new services to evidence of effectiveness. In addition to permitting insurers to avoid paying for treatments considered to be ineffective, the discretionary capacity to set coverage policy could also be used to extract pricing concessions from manufacturers when the evidence for comparative efficacy is more ambiguous. As discussed in chapter 2, success in implementing such a policy, public or private, will require significant efforts to build a solid base of evidence about the comparative efficacy of treatment alternatives.

Second, insurance programs can vary the out-of-pocket costs that beneficiaries face when considering choices among available diagnostic and treatment options. Drug benefit programs, for example, often use tiered co-payments, under which beneficiaries face substantially higher co-payments if they elect to use nonpreferred products. The preferred product in these circumstances is designated today on the basis of purely economic considerations, for example, the willingness of the manufacturer to offer deep discounts in exchange for favorable formulary placement. However, such incentives could also be used to influence patient and provider decisionmaking so that decisions are based on clinical criteria, including comparative efficacy. Such efforts are currently very limited, as the evidence base to support such clinical distinctions is sparse. Moreover, it is difficult to make such decisions on a wholesale basis, because a therapy that proves superior for the vast majority of patients may still prove inferior to available alternatives for a limited subset of patients.

Third, insurance programs can condition coverage for a particular service for a particular patient on prospective review of the appropriateness of the service before the service is rendered. Although this approach has long been used to deter unnecessary elective hospitalizations, traditional insurance programs and managed care plans have extended such prior authorization programs to costly services, such as advanced technology imaging procedures. However, there may be limits to expanding this approach. Such gatekeeper programs were an important driver of the backlash against tightly controlled managed care systems in the late 1990s. In addition, subsequent evaluations by the health benefits management industry have demonstrated that prior authorization may be truly cost effective only for very high cost items such as extended inpatient stays.

Looking forward, our assessment is that the only hope for the adoption of administrative measures or pricing signals to promote serious cost containment lies in investment in developing research and policy processes that the public—as well as providers and patients—can regard as evidence based, not politically based.

Facilitation and Forbearance

Apart from their role as stewards of public-sector insurance systems, what role should public policymakers play in easing the transition to serious cost containment?

As suggested above, the primary barrier to evidence-based decision-making is the lack of rigorous evidence about the comparative effectiveness of most of what is done in medicine. While this has long been true regarding clinical issues, separate and apart from considerations of cost, it is equally true of evidence that would be helpful in assessing trade-offs between comparative efficacy and cost. To enable serious cost containment, it is essential to make substantial progress on building the evidence base.

We believe that the public sector has a critical role to play in facilitating the development of this evidence base. As noted in chapter 2, the government can be an important actor by funding required research and coordinating this research to ensure that private-sector efforts are directed toward the most pressing cost management problems. We are aware that many affected constituencies will perceive an active conflict between the government's role as a sponsor of insurance plans and its role as research facilitator. As long as there are federally funded insurance systems, we do not believe that this can be helped. If serious cost containment is to succeed, government as facilitator must fund this research and government as payer must use it. To be successful in this dual role, government must become far more transparent than it is today regarding the use of clinical evidence in making coverage and payment policy decisions. The key to serious cost containment, we believe, lies in the creation of a process that encourages the generation of balanced, scientifically rigorous research to inform decisionmaking about coverage and reimbursement policies. If that process, in turn, facilitates transformation of the public and private health financing system into a mechanism to internalize the incentives that will promote cost-conscious care for all Americans, then the public's long-term interest in health care reform will have been finally satisfied.

Notes

1. This section draws heavily on previously published material. See Judith Feder, "Crowd-out and the Politics of Health Reform," *Journal of Law, Medicine & Ethics* 32, no. 3 (2004): 461–64.

2. Timothy S. Jost, *Disentitlement? The Threats Facing Our Public Health-Care Programs and a Rights-Based Response* (Oxford University Press, 2003); Jennifer Klein, *For All These Rights: Business, Labor, and the Shaping of America's Public-Private Welfare State* (Princeton University Press, 2003); Jacob Hacker, *The Divided Welfare State* (Cambridge University Press, 2002).

3. Medicaid also supplements Medicare for its low-income elderly and the later-added disabled beneficiaries and provides long-term care to those who satisfy eligibility and financial requirements.

4. For data on the uninsured, see Kaiser Commission on Medicaid and the Uninsured, *Health Insurance Coverage in America, 2002 Data Update* (Washington: Henry J. Kaiser Family Foundation, 2003).

5. Robert Stevens and Rosemary Stevens, *Welfare Medicine in America: A Case Study of Medicaid* (New York: Free Press, 1974).

6. Expansions over the years have nevertheless moved somewhat closer to workers, by covering children of lower-income workers; pregnant women in working two-parent households; and persons with disabilities who could return to the workplace with support. States have the option to cover parents (fathers as well as mothers), but in most states, parents earning the minimum wage have too much income to qualify for Medicaid. And except in a few states that operate their Medicaid programs as special federally sanctioned demonstrations that waive traditional Medicaid eligibility restrictions, federal law, today as in 1965, does not extend Medicaid eligibility to low-income adults who are not parents of dependent children.

7. Cristina Boccuti and Marilyn Moon, "Comparing Medicare and Private Insurers: Growth Rates in Spending over Three Decades," *Health Affairs* 22, no. 2 (2003): 230–37.

8. Todd Gilmer and Richard Kronick, "It's The Premiums Stupid: Projections of the Uninsured through 2013," *Health Affairs* web exclusive, April 5, 2005: W5-143–W5-151. Todd Gilmer and Richard Kronick, "Calm before the Storm: Expected Increase in the Number of Uninsured Americans," *Health Affairs* 20, no. 6 (2001): 207–10.

9. Kaiser and HRET, *Employer Health Benefits, 2006* (Washington: Henry J. Kaiser Family Foundation, Health Research and Educational Trust, September 26, 2006).

10. The Congressional Budget Office ultimately judged this employer mandate to constitute a "tax," though whether the public perceived it as such is an open question.

11. But see note 6, supra.

12. Medicare savings were dedicated to the proposal's prescription drug and long-term care benefits.

13. Although the Congressional Budget Office did not find these and other projected savings entirely sufficient to finance the program, its estimates came close (and indeed were achievable with modest adjustments to some of the proposed benefits and subsidies).

14. Robert T. Blendon, Mollyanne Brodie, and John Benson, "What Happened to Americans' Support for the Clinton Health Plan," *Health Affairs* 14, no. 2 (1995): 7–23.

15. The Health Insurance Association of America subsequently merged with the American Association of Health Plans to form America's Health Insurance Plans.

16. Andrew Kohut and others, *The 2004 Political Landscape: Evenly Divided and Increasingly Polarized* (Washington: Pew Research Center for the People and the Press, November 5, 2003) (people-press.org/reports/display.php3?ReportID=196).

17. John Breaux, "Ceasefire on Health Care: A Centrist's Approach to Reform," commentary (New York: Commonwealth Fund, March 2006) (www.cmwf.org/publications/publications_show.htm?doc_id=362364).

18. A concise, balanced narrative can be found in Jill Quadagno, "Why the United States Has No National Health Insurance: Stakeholder Mobilization against the Welfare State, 1945–1996," *Journal of Health and Social Behavior* 45 (extra issue, December 2004): 25–44.

19. Congressional Budget Office, *Background Material on the Catastrophic Drug Insurance Program* (July 1989).

20. Jill Quadagno, "Why the United States Has No National Health Insurance."

21. Throughout the 1990s, however, a significant number of beneficiaries received a prescription drug benefit—frequently at no incremental premium—by electing to enroll in a Medicare managed care option.

22. Under the commission's charter, a supermajority of voting members was required to formally report recommendations. Although a majority of members voted to adopt the commission recommendation, heavy lobbying by interests concerned about the commission's proposed policy caused the commission to fail to reach the required supermajority—by one vote.

23. National Bipartisan Commission on the Future of Medicare, *Building a Better Medicare for Today and Tomorrow* (Washington, March 16, 1999).

24. "Remaking Medicare," *NewsHour with Jim Lehrer,* Public Broadcasting System, March 17, 1999.

25. The commission policy was commonly labeled with the names of the bipartisan cochairs of the commission—Senator John Breaux (D-La.) and House Ways and Means Committee chairman Bill Thomas (R-Calif.).

26. The most complete account of the policy history traced in this section is contained in Thomas R. Oliver, Philip R. Lee, Helene L. Lipton, "A Political History of Medicare and Prescription Drug Coverage," *Milbank Quarterly* 82, no. 2 (2004): 283–354.

27. While Republicans controlled Congress during the early stage of the debate from 1999 to 2002, the Democrats achieved working control of the Senate in 2003–04 when Senator Jim Jeffords of Vermont announced his conversion to Independent status and his willingness to vote with the Democrats to organize the Senate.

28. Although hundreds of other provisions came together from both the Senate and House sides to ride the train of this moving legislation, they were unrelated to the central debate over the structure of the drug benefit.

29. The final provisions on cost containment—Title VIII of P. L. 108-391—substituted procedural notice of fiscal stresses in the system for any attempt to actually change the benefit entitlement.

30. Donald W. Moran, "Whence and Whither Health Insurance? A Revisionist History," *Health Affairs* 24, no. 6 (2005): 1415–425.

8

Building Public Support for Slowing the Growth of Health Care Spending

STUART M. BUTLER

The task of moving from policy proposal to successful legislation means navigating the waters of public opinion that influences practical politics. This is true of all areas of policy, of course, but health care waters are especially turbulent. Health care is intensely personal and costly for families, and even small policy changes have potentially huge financial implications for them as well as other stakeholders. If successful ways of addressing the health spending challenge are to be devised, it is critical to reflect on the underlying values and moral choices associated with any policy approach. The wise policymaker will thus consider policy refinements or pursue policy options that might make proposals more compatible with the underlying values of Americans—or at least to pose initiatives in ways that force the public to consider the moral trade-offs involved.

The Challenge of Achieving Health Care Spending Reform

Achieving public policy goals in health care is particularly difficult because of the way in which Americans think about health policy proposals. As

Daniel Yankelovich has explained in his classic work on how people make policy decisions, people go through stages in deciding what should be done about an issue.[1] These stages range from focusing on the issue currently on the "radar screen" for most people and acquiring urgency, to weighing choices and trade-offs, and finally to making decisions about those choices. The problem with health care—more than most other major issues—is that while Americans certainly think of health care and health care costs (more precisely, the costs they face) as a critical issue, there is enormous confusion, wishful thinking, internal contradiction, and emotion entangled in the way people evaluate health policy proposals. People tend to look at health proposals from a personal and financial viewpoint but also in terms of basic values and perspectives—such as rights, fairness, risk, and obligation. These feelings are typically not well-articulated or often even understood by those who hold them, which is why traditional public opinion polling on health can be so contradictory and misleading. But because people are likely to react to health proposals in this way, careful consideration of the value choices triggered by approaches to the health spending challenge is critically important.

The chapters in this volume discuss three general goals, each of which has important practical implications for Americans and hence for the way they are likely to respond to specific proposals. One goal is to improve the efficiency with which Americans spend health dollars—getting better value for money. Improving efficiency might seem noncontroversial. But as discussed below, the meaning of "value" is often intensely subjective. For example, what seems like unnecessary small talk to a doctor may seem like caring, personal attention to the patient.[2] So what is deemed to be value in health care spending decisions, and who makes those decisions, is critical to public acceptance of those decisions.

A second goal is to limit expenditures, through incentives or controls. This goal enters the picture because even if society could agree on what constitutes efficiency, and on steps that would improve it, growth in spending would not necessarily moderate. For example, if people have a pent-up demand for medical services, and their spending is constrained only by their acceptable out-of-pocket cost, then improving value for money while retaining today's subsidies and incentives would lead people to increase total consumption of services for the same level of out-of-pocket spending, not to reduce their spending. More direct control of spending or changed incentives would still have to be introduced to cause a restraint in spending growth. The tools available to do that, such as market incentives or expenditure controls, each require tough decisions that raise deeper issues.

But there is a third goal, or perhaps a group of goals, that is interwoven in the other two—the goal of fairness, or equity. While important to the policymaker, of course, the idea of fairness is central to whether typical Americans will accept a policy. How people visualize "fairness" is associated with deeply held values and is often subjective, making broad public acceptance of a plan to improve efficiency or hold down costs all the more difficult. Many Americans see access to some level of health care as a right of citizenship and balk at any action that would seem to contradict that notion of right. Many also place great weight on the idea of equity in health care, leading them to resist steps that seem to treat similar people in different ways. Fairness affects the way people think about obligations and responsibilities involved in health care; how these should be distributed between individuals, employers, and different layers of society; and who should make these decisions. Fairness also affects the way people respond to the degree of economic risk they consider reasonable to expect a family—or the taxpayer—to shoulder. And fairness influences the degree to which Americans think government or employers should honor promises made long ago, even if those promises conflict with commercial viability or other urgent spending or tax goals.

Improving Efficiency while Achieving Equity

While everybody would agree with the general proposition that it is good to improve efficiency, there is intense debate about what constitutes efficiency in the case of health care. To an economist, efficiency in health care means allocating the level and combination of services in a way that produces the greatest medical benefits with the fewest economic resources.[3] But while seeking to be efficient, policymakers also must seek to distribute health services in a way that maximizes the nation's collective preferences, recognizing people's notions of equity and fairness.

Several difficulties and conflicts arise when policymakers actually try to do this. There are what one might call technical arguments. Even if efficiency is considered simply as achieving a specific medical outcome (such as removing a kidney stone or curing a cancer) with the least economic resources, and even if all the externalities involved could be captured, Antos and Rivlin explain in chapter 2 that there are still uncertainties and disputes about what approach actually produces the best medical outcome.

Another difficulty is far more intractable. Even assuming that it is possible to agree that certain techniques will maximize efficiency in achieving specific medical outcomes, there is wide and subjective disagreement on what constitutes the "benefit" or "value" of a particular procedure for a particular patient. For example, is it good value for money to carry out a double knee replacement on an 85-year-old man? The answer depends on what is meant by "value" and who is doing the measuring. Putting aside for the moment the issue of who is paying the bill and comparing cost, different people will have very different assessments of value. The patient probably has a very different vision of benefit than an insurance benefits manager or the director of the Office of Management and Budget. And a lifelong walker likely will place a different value on the replacement than would a couch potato. So two seemingly identical patients with identical prognoses might envision very different benefits from the operation because value is highly subjective. Economist David Cutler points out that even though the perceived value of a health improvement is heavily subjective, some tools are available to help quantify people's subjective valuations.[4] For example, the additional years of active life typically associated with a procedure can be measured. But trying to design policies that take account of the wide variation of valuations is a daunting task. Imagine designing and enforcing a bureaucratic regulation to ensure that the 85-year-old walker got knee replacement and the couch potato did not. If the way cases are actually resolved and resource decisions made seems unjust to politically influential segments of the population, achieving reforms to rein in spending becomes extremely difficult.

Private versus Social Perceptions of Value and Efficiency

Some would argue that allowing markets to resolve these subjective value-for-money decisions is the most logical and value-neutral allocation system because markets place the locus of control in the hands of the user of medical services. Surveys show that the personal choice in health that accompanies markets is a strongly held value. And when individuals have more responsibility for spending resources, the argument goes, they have a greater incentive to calculate whether a particular array of services, including new technologies, delivers the best value for the money they can spend. When Americans buy cars or computers out of their own resources, for instance, the purchasers weigh the cost of technologies to enhance performance or safety against the benefit they perceive they will receive—including unique, subjective value.

But some analysts raise cautions about reliance on markets. In a technologically complex area like health, one natural concern is that individuals are not well equipped to identify the goods and services that will most efficiently deliver the value they seek. As Wilensky emphasizes in chapter 3, good and available information about outcomes and costs, among other things, is essential if consumer-driven decisions are to be efficient. Moreover, in health as in other decisions involving significant and technically complex decisions, such as buying a house or picking a college for one's child, consumers often turn to "agents" to help them process information and make a decision. Agents not only have to be knowledgeable; the consumer must also trust the agent to offer advice or make a decision in line with the consumer's values.

Even putting aside these concerns, using markets as a policy tool to achieve economic efficiency in health care raises several additional issues. One is whether a market is transparent, in the sense of the patient decisionmaker taking into full account the cost of resources involved when comparing subjective benefits with costs. As Antos and Rivlin explain in chapter 2 and Ginsburg in chapter 6, that comparison is heavily skewed in favor of choosing more health service for millions of Americans in the private sector because of the tax treatment of health insurance when an employer organizes the insurance. Even though the insurance is in reality a cost to the employee, in the form of forgone cash income, the cost is veiled to the employee and so encourages inefficient decisions and higher expenditures than would occur if an individual compared (subjective) value with the true cost. Several proposals in earlier chapters that are designed to improve efficiency by sharpening market incentives raise these issues of transparency and social goals. One aim of proposals to reform the tax treatment of health insurance, for example, is to improve transparency and present people with a clearer comparison of cost and perceived benefit when making a health decision.

SOCIAL VALUE. A deeper issue is whether improving an individual's perceived value for money would actually capture the full meaning of efficiency. In particular, it is open to question whether an individual's personal, subjective view of value for money should be the determinant of efficiency in all cases, even if the person were to have full information and complete control of resources and unerringly maximized medical outcomes. Can society allow people to fail to vaccinate their children against measles, for example, just because they personally do not value the protection?

The complication is social value. Let us say that as a national or state community we have concluded that there are broader social values related to health care that normal markets do not recognize and that encouraging more (or less) spending on health by certain people helps to achieve a social goal. For example, a social goal might be that as a "membership right" of society, all Americans should be able to obtain an adequate level of health care ("adequate" being a political decision, not an objective one); that access to good health care, like high rates of home ownership, is part of the American Dream. Such a goal could lead a community to decide collectively that subsidizing private spending on health care is a social good, and it might do so not just through spending programs but also by tax preferences (as the federal government does for both health care and home ownership).

But a decision to subsidize health care also raises the issue of whether the community is concerned about the type and volume of care that is purchased with the subsidy. If funds are transferred from the wider community to an individual so that society can achieve the social goal of a certain standard of health care for every person, it is reasonable for the community to have some say in the level and type of care the person receives with the transferred funds or tax preference.[5] It is also reasonable to argue that the higher the proportion of spending on health that comes from this community funding, as opposed to the individual's own funds, the greater the case for the community to determine what constitutes value in the services provided. By this argument, the use of public funds means the broader community's view of the efficiency of technology, services, and procedures (such as a knee replacement) can trump the individual's view of efficiency at least to some degree. This line of argument is used to justify some level of required benefit package when public funds are involved. The same logic for a benefit design applies to other services where public funds are used, either directly to pay providers or through vouchers, such as in housing or education.

VALUE IN PUBLIC AND PRIVATE COVERAGE. The case for the community having a voice in determining value and efficiency is perhaps strongest in Medicaid and other programs for low-income individuals, where all or almost all of the funding comes from the public. In these programs it is reasonable to argue for procedures to assign a value to a certain service based on the goals of social policy and to include or exclude the service from a benefit package. In a federal-state program like Medicaid, there is of course the complicating issue of who can speak for the wider community since different streams of public funds are involved. But there is also a strong case for a wider community's voice to be heard in Medicare. To be sure, the beneficiary contributes payroll contributions, premiums, and out-of-pocket spending. But the program also includes a huge contribution from the general taxpayer. It does this explicitly in Part B, which primarily covers physician costs and is not funded by the Medicare payroll tax. But it also does so implicitly for the whole program because of unfunded Medicare obligations.

Social objectives as a factor in measuring value and efficiency are not confined to public sector programs, however. To be sure, a compelling general case can be made for saying that when people spend their own money on health care, they should be the sole arbiters of value and efficiency (an example might be expensive Botox treatments for wrinkles). Yet to the extent that tax policy is specifically designed to alter decisions by transferring funds and subsidizing health services through focused tax relief and credits, the wider community can reasonably demand at least some say in how the transferred money is used. Consider proposals to limit or cap the tax exclusion for employer-sponsored insurance while creating a refundable tax credit for moderate and lower-income individuals. Proponents argue that this approach would directly increase economic efficiency by exposing upper-income individuals to more of the true cost of coverage by reducing the tax subsidy from other taxpayers. In addition, a refundable credit would offset the cost of health care for lower-income workers and induce greater utilization of health care compared with unsubsidized goods and services. A community could decide that this result achieves a social goal of greater equity in access to health care. It could also conclude that the tax credit would lead to more efficient use of public finances, by reducing revenue loss in the tax system and by inducing lower-income households to seek timely care rather than ending up in emergency rooms with more severe health problems or in expensive public programs.

As noted in earlier chapters, the current tax system provides a large benefit to upper-income employees, because employer-sponsored health benefits are free of all taxes. So a tax credit/exclusion cap reform would even out the community-financed benefit. Moreover, since a tax exclusion or tax credit is intended to achieve a public purpose, the argument can be made that specific benefits and coverage requirements can and should be a condition of tax relief for private plans to achieve the public purpose of access to a particular level and type of health care. Some use this line of argument to propose that tax credits should be restricted in use to certain sources of plans, such as employer coverage or state pools. Still, even where the argument is accepted in principle, the acceptable degree of community control is fiercely debated.

Why Limit the Growth of Spending?

However one decides to resolve questions of value and efficiency, improving efficiency is not the same as reining in total spending. Society can have low or high efficiency at any amount of spending. And while efficiency improvements likely will moderate the growth of health spending—although the degree is disputed—the authors of various chapters note that the total amount of health care spending is heavily driven by the incentives and commitments built into the system. So if the growth of health spending is to slow, policymakers must revisit those incentives and commitments and ponder the implications of making any changes.

Should policymakers even be trying to reduce the growth of health care costs? It might be argued that if efficiency has been improved in an agreeable way, then policymakers should not be concerned about the amount Americans spend on health care, either in dollar terms or as a proportion of the national economy. After all, society does not tend to worry about the proportion of the national output that is devoted to housing, cars, or movies. So is there really such a thing as a correct or ideal level of health spending? If a rising share of GDP for health care was no longer considered inherently troubling, at least a paradox would be resolved: faster rates of building and employment growth in family or commercial construction are trumpeted as good for the economy and the American future, yet announcements of faster hospital building or employment are greeted with alarm. Moreover, there might be sound reasons for health spending to be increasing as a proportion of GDP. For example, as the population ages, one would expect a service disproportionately consumed by older Americans to push up health spending. As average Americans become richer, one would also expect an increased preference for spending on improvements to health relative to other uses of money, leading to a higher proportion of national income devoted to health.

A distinction might be drawn between spending growth in the private sector and in the public sector. If people are spending their private resources on health care in ways that give them satisfaction, even if doctors and some economists say those ways are unnecessary and wasteful, should policymakers really be concerned? Provided that policymakers ensure that private markets are working fairly and regulated efficiently, it could be said that policymakers should not worry about the level and preferences of private health spending any more than spending levels on movies, vacations, or iPods. At the same time, one might argue that public spending on health reflects public preferences, and so policymakers would be right to focus on spending levels in the public sector.

As previous chapters indicate, even if this distinction is accepted in principle, there are public policy reasons to be concerned about two things when direct subsidies or tax preferences are involved: the level of public subsidy associated with the extra health spending induced, and the type of spending induced.

Certainly in the public sector, the government has an obligation to consider the costs of pursuing health policy goals. It must consider spending on health care objectives in relation to other, competing public goals, as well as the cumulative economic effects of government spending. As discussed below, this raises the issue of how and whether long-term promises can be kept. Should the government modify public programs in which it has made promises that cannot be honored in the future without an unacceptable diversion of funds from other programs, future tax or debt burdens to finance the promises, or slower economic growth?

Consider once again spending in the private sector. It would be hard for most Americans to accept a general proposition that the government should seek to restrict people's ability in the private sector to spend their own money on their own health care—or their employer from doing so using part of their compensation. This would be true even if that money is spent on health services the vast majority would not choose. But when public funds are entwined with private dollars, or when a certain private expenditure is encouraged with tax relief, the equation changes and there is a reason for concern. The generous tax treatment of employer-sponsored health insurance artificially skews private preferences for health care compared with other goods and services, boosting health spending beyond the level that would otherwise occur. It becomes legitimate for the community to be concerned about private sector health spending when subsidies or tax relief is involved. The argument is not that the government should limit private spending on health care, but that the government should not subsidize artificially high private spending—at least by those with higher incomes.

Thinking about the Sanctity of Promises

The entitlement status in the federal budget of programs like Medicare and Medicaid conveys a critically important moral dimension. These entitlements represent long-term promises to deliver a defined benefit without the limitations of a normal budget. Hence proposals to reduce the scope of the benefits, or the eligibility or funding levels, are widely interpreted by Americans as reneging on a solemn promise. So it is unlikely that proposals to curb spending on these programs will be politically successful unless proponents can reshape the understanding of health care promises in the minds of Americans.

Entitlements versus Discretionary Commitments

The challenge for policymakers seeking to curb health entitlement programs is to persuade Americans that it is reasonable and fair to balance these promises against the cost of other legitimate goals and implicit promises made to other worthy groups. For if the promises are seen in isolation, and the true cost hidden, Americans are not faced with a moral trade-off and resist proposals that seem to weaken a solemn commitment.

If people are even to consider a trade-off between health care commitments and other promises, they must first, of course, accept that circumstances require a trade-off. Surveys indicate that Americans today generally do not readily accept that premise.[6] Beside the typical affliction of wishful thinking—that all goals and desires could be achieved if "waste" were eliminated—resistance to the idea of a trade-off also occurs because the budget process allows politicians to avoid discussing difficult long-term budget trade-offs. While the annual Medicare Trustees report lays great emphasis on the long-term unfunded obligations of Medicare, the federal budget considered by Congress ignores the present value of long-term commitments, considering only the five-year or at most ten-year spending scenarios. So lawmakers have little incentive to make difficult decisions to curb future spending obligations or to avoid politically attractive new programs with immediate benefits but costs that mushroom over time. The absence of long-term spending consequences in the budget helps explain why Congress in 2003 enacted a multitrillion dollar Medicare drug bill while claiming it was clamping down on spending.

Changing the Budget Process

A necessary condition for public discussion of moral and spending trade-offs is to make the budget trade-offs more transparent and public. One small but critical step would be to amend the budget process to include a present-value measure of long-term entitlement obligations and special tax preferences in the annual budget process and to incorporate changes in the present value into the annual budget resolution. Several proposals introduced in Congress would incorporate such a change.[7] This change would at least bring long-term commitments into the limelight of the

annual budget. To be sure, there are legitimate disputes over the methodology and accuracy of estimating the present value of future health spending. But this is a case where even a crude estimate would sharply improve
the nature of the public discussion.

Building on greater transparency, a more radical step would make the
trade-offs between health programs and other goals even more visible
and less avoidable by requiring annual federal budgets to comply with a
long-term spending and financing plan. This step would convert Medicare
and Medicaid from entitlements to discretionary programs and set a long-
range budget. This would end the preferential entitlement status of the
programs and force decisions to be made regularly and on a more equal
footing between health promises and other promises (such as promises to
protect the nation or to educate the young), and between the burden of
these spending programs and the economic costs of taxation. Recognizing that planning for retirement requires some certainty over time, a discretionary budget for Medicare might be included prominently in the
budget for, say, a thirty-year period, along with a financing budget that
would adequately cover obligations. This long-term spending and financing plan would be adjusted regularly in light of such things as changes in
technology and demographics. The five- or ten-year budgets enacted by
Congress would have to comply with this longer-term budget plan. The
long-term plan, as well as the shorter-term budgets, could be linked to
some degree to underlying medical costs in order to provide a level of certainty and protection. Indeed an indexed or voucherized budget can be
designed to set the financial risk at any point along a spectrum between
the community holding the whole risk (a defined benefit entitlement) to
the individual holding the entire risk (an "arbitrary" fixed budget). Whatever the fine-tuning, there would be a real, limited budget that could be
revisited periodically and adjusted in light of economic conditions and
new priorities.

Changing entitlement health programs such as Medicare into discretionary programs would effectively give these programs the same budget
status as the SCHIP program. To keep spending within the budget limit,
Congress would periodically have to take specific steps, such as changing
eligibility rules, altering the covered benefits, implementing greater
means-testing, or adjusting payments to providers. Some have suggested

a "trigger" mechanism that would implement automatic adjustments in eligibility or provider payments if the budget is exceeded.[8] To be sure, designing and enforcing a health spending trigger is no easy task. Reducing payments in Medicare is a form of price control, for instance, and would cause providers to try to game the trigger by increasing volume or reclassifying procedures. And triggers based on fee payments to doctors or changes in eligibility can be so politically sensitive that they are reversed. Nonetheless, for the policymaking process the prospect of a trigger, much like Benjamin Franklin's reflection on the prospect of hanging, can concentrate the mind—and lead to a program redesign to address the budget requirements.

Forcing Americans to confront a trade-off between health entitlement spending and other goals is a necessary condition for spending control, but it is not a sufficient condition. To agree to such a major change in spending, Americans also would have to be persuaded of at least two things. One is the proposition that it is unfair for promises made to current and future retirees to trump commitments to other worthy groups, such as children or soldiers, irrespective of the economic conditions or the accepted importance of those other needs. Another, in the case of the funding obligations for Medicare, is the proposition that it is unfair simply to expect future generations to have to fully honor commitments they were not necessarily even a party to making—or at least that intergenerational commitments are renegotiable.

Contemplating Risk

Making the case for limiting the growth in health care entitlement expenditures is especially difficult because risk is central to the discussion. Revisiting the implicit social contract between the generations and between health commitments and other social obligations means balancing financial risks associated with health.

When it comes to their health, Americans have shown in their voting patterns and insurance decisions that they want the financial risk associated with an accident or illness to be minimized. Yet their very concept of risk in health is different from that in other spheres, and it has been changing. In health, for instance, there seems to be a quest not only to avoid wide variations in personal spending but also to achieve the goal of reducing one's personal spending while constantly increasing one's level of care. Detroit workers with pink slips, however, and looming obligations in Medicare, indicate how illusory that goal is becoming. Moreover, the term "risk" traditionally referred to things that might or might not happen—an accident, a dread disease, or falling into such poverty that one could not afford the minimum acceptable level of health care. These were the unexpected health concerns for which private and social insurance was intended. But today there is an additional form of risk that has shaped Americans' view of risk in health care and their attitude to health programs—the "risk" that in the future they might not be able to obtain the constantly improving health services associated with the good life. Things can be done in health care today—expensively—that were virtually unthinkable a few decades ago, and they can improve and extend life to a degree that most previous generations would not have even imagined, let alone thought of as a right to be guaranteed by society. The fear that in the future one may not share in this presumed right is at the heart of the risk of unfulfilled expectations; a product, says journalist Robert Samuelson, of the "postaffluent society."[9]

Americans plan for this expanded view of health risks either by reducing them (such as avoiding certain lifestyles), saving in advance, or insuring against them. The last strategy spreads the risk by sharing it in some collective fashion through private insurance, social insurance, or programs supported through general taxation. Private insurance spreads risk across a voluntary association of those people who choose to purchase insurance—although in tax-advantaged employer-sponsored insurance the employer effectively controls the purchase decision and the portion of the employee's compensation devoted to insurance, so the term "choose" is somewhat illusory.

By their very design, however, social insurance and direct spending programs do not distribute a random financial risk across a normal insurance group of individuals; they assign the risk to a community, usually the national community. But when the financial risk to one individual or small community is reduced in this way, the risk to another individual or community increases. Thus entitlements in the public sector, like defined benefit plans in private companies, do reduce the financial risk for the beneficiary, but they increase the financial risk to the wider community that is obligated to finance the entitlement. So proposals to rein in spending in these programs force Americans to consider what constitutes a fair distribution of financial risk. In particular, policymakers must consider how Americans will react to policy changes that alter the relative risks shouldered by health beneficiaries and the beneficiaries of other programs, by the federal government and the states, and by different generations.

THE BALANCE OF RISK BETWEEN GROUPS. Health entitlements and other health spending reduce the financial risk for beneficiaries but increase the risk for groups with needs that must compete for funds and generally for groups that are dependent on discretionary programs. For example, Eugene Steuerle has drawn attention to the way in which middle-class entitlements, especially Medicare, are relentlessly crowding out funds for children's programs. This crowding out will accelerate as the baby boom generation retires.[10] If Americans were asked explicitly if they found this trend acceptable they might consider spending reforms. But the budget process clouds the picture. As discussed earlier, if policymakers are to achieve policy decisions on health spending that reflect the balance that Americans want to achieve between competing social goals and the underlying values they represent, then the budget process must make such trade-offs much more transparent.

FEDERAL AND STATE RISK REDUCTION. A policy designed to reduce federal costs in health entitlements—that is, to reduce the financial risk to current and future taxpayers—also requires consideration of the financial risk to states and even lower levels of government that have a legal or moral obligation (under pressure from voters) to maintain acceptable levels of care. One suggested way to reduce the risk to states is to give them greater flexibility and incentives to find more efficient ways to design and deliver services, and the legal power to adjust eligibility or services for some categories of beneficiary. This can be done through waivers and block grants. However, advocates of Medicaid and other programs for low-income Americans understandably worry that retrenchment at the federal level means benefit and eligibility changes that may insulate state coffers while shifting the risk down to vulnerable beneficiaries of the programs. The complaint from advocates is that, all other things equal, this flexibility means higher out-of-pocket payments, reduced availability of services, and even reduced eligibility for individuals whom average Americans generally want to help.

Is there a way to address risk-shifting between levels of government that might better address the concern that the financial risk and burden on the poor would be excessive? Perhaps this can be done by edging toward an acceptance of tiering in health care for those in need. Based on the pattern of federal and state legislation over the years, society does seem to be striving to assure all residents that they can count on some minimum level and scope of health care from the community if they cannot afford it themselves. But Americans also seem to take the view that beyond that minimum it is appropriate for states to vary the level of benefits and categories of beneficiaries as reflected in the resources and the social values of their citizens. So there seems to be a distinction drawn between a national community obligation and smaller communities in which preferences and capacities shape any additional obligation. This sense of tiered obligation is already enshrined in the mandatory and optional populations in Medicaid and SCHIP.

As we consider how states might adapt to the financial risk associated with reining in federal spending and the concern it raises for beneficiaries, perhaps the federal government's role should be clarified in light of the way Americans look at spreading risk and obligations between different levels of community. The approach might be to clarify in statute both the national goals of federal-state programs and the national protections that must apply to beneficiary groups, but give states much wider flexibility than today in how they organize health services to achieve those goals.[11] It is important to recognize, of course, that the principle of tiering means that beyond a minimum national set of benefits and eligibility for public programs in America, it has to be acceptable for needy individuals to receive different levels and types of care than do better-off Americans. These differences reflect not just local (that is, state) financial capacities, but also differing views of the proper balance among social commitments to health care and to other goals such as education or housing.

RISKS TO INDIVIDUALS. However society tries to sort out the financial risks to different communities associated with restraining total federal health spending, experience shows it is very difficult to get public support unless Americans feel that ultimately the financial risks to individuals are handled reasonably and fairly.

That sense of fairness depends on the nature of the risk and the individuals at risk. For instance, Americans typically feel that those who "play by the rules" and have tried to plan for the future deserve more protection than those who have not. And most think it is especially unfair to change the rules on someone who has tried to plan but does not easily have the ability to adapt to changes in a program. The capacity of a person to plan for change or adapt to it is central to the public's sense of fairness about spending controls. The pattern of legislation in recent years indicates a strong public resistance to budget reductions in Medicare that would significantly affect current retirees or those nearing retirement but some openness to higher costs, such as through income-testing, on more affluent seniors.

More ambivalence occurs in the case of the Medicaid population. A strong desire to help those who fall on hard times is balanced against a tendency to view many on Medicaid as having more generous health care protection than most who work and are modestly paid. Moreover, the recent pattern of state Medicaid changes suggests that the public's commitment to low-income working-age people and their children who are needy is seen, rightly or wrongly, as more limited and temporary than its obligation, say, to the elderly. The Medicaid commitment is seen as dependent on the community's available resources—with the obligation to children more strongly felt than to parents and especially to single adults without children. At the same time, the strong commitment to those who are reaching retirement is broadly perceived as a higher-order promise to repay those who have contributed to their health benefits— Americans think of Medicare benefits as something people earn and that reducing earned benefits is unfair.

Rationing

The discussion in the previous chapters points to two broad approaches intended to curb spending within the context of public perceptions of fairness. One is to place greater control of the allocation and pricing of health services in the hands of government. The aim in this case is to allocate resources according to a community-wide sense of fairness and efficiency. The other approach is to invest control mainly in the hands of individual users of services, with markets as the tool to allocate resources. The aim in this case is to give individuals the ability to allocate resources in ways that maximize their own preferences. Both involve rationing, in the simple sense that total resources (private combined with public contributions) are less than the demand, and both raise issues about control in the context of risk.

Americans flinch from the term "rationing," in the sense of government officials making decisions over who will or will not receive particular medical services. But then they also flinch from the idea that medical service decisions should be made on the basis of who can afford to pay a premium or out-of-pocket price. In fact, rationing in the sense of denying services according to some criterion (perhaps by price, perhaps by a formula to determine "need") is implicit in every system of allocating any resource.

Each general rationing technique raises different values and ethical concerns in people's minds. Rationing by explicit denial of access, for instance, raises the issue of who in the community should make these decisions and on what moral basis? Rationing by payment to service providers, either in the public or private sector, raises additional concerns. For example, should health providers be the ones who must make rationing decisions when their costs exceed their payments from the government or insurers?[12] Conversely, should the high salaries of doctors relative to other professions (compared with other countries) be considered sacrosanct? Furthermore, rationing by price at the point of consumption, through deductibles and co-payments, raises the general question of whether ability to pay should be the determinant of access to all care, or perhaps only to access for certain categories of care.

Devising successful policies to slow the growth of health expenditures actually requires policymakers to consider how people view these different forms of rationing—not just how mechanically efficient the forms are, but how they conform to people's sense of values and fairness.

The public's willingness to accept rationing in the form of government agencies deciding whether specific items are covered services depends in large part on whether people have confidence in the way the political process makes these decisions. One possible way of reducing these concerns is to make coverage decisions as objective as possible, by reducing the perception that decisions are the result of provider lobbyists or other pressures. Oregon sought to resolve these concerns by ranking services according to the medical evidence on their cost-effectiveness and using public meetings and dialogs to build acceptance among Oregonians for eliminating less effective services in order to stay within the budget. Meanwhile Canada and the United Kingdom have procedures to regulate the introduction of new technology into their systems. In the United States, some have proposed a "Benefits Board" of medical experts to revise the Medicare package, in place of Congress legislating benefits in an atmosphere of lobbying and gridlock. The proposed board would periodically recommend the most cost-effective and modern benefits package for a budget, and Congress would have to enact or reject the package without amendment.[13]

However, these seemingly objective approaches trigger two general concerns. The first is the issue of subjective value raised earlier in the discussion of efficiency, namely, that the value judgments of a panel charged with assessing the benefit of a procedure necessarily will often differ sharply from those who are subject to its decisions. Ranking disputes in Oregon often centered on these value judgments. So in its Medicaid reform plan of the early 1990s, the state sought to address this by incorporating a series of public meetings to gauge opinion and refine its ranking of services.[14] The second and related concern is the fear that a remote panel of "faceless" individuals will make mechanical decisions and cannot be reasoned with—the worry that lies at the heart of the widespread antipathy to insurance companies and particularly to managed care. Unless and until explicit rationing system procedures in public programs are perceived to engage those affected and to be flexible, it is likely that Americans will resist the idea of politicians or bureaucracies directly limiting their care.

To be sure, the more common form of rationing in the United States is not by directly allowing or disallowing access to care, but by regulating the payment for care. Private markets do this through pricing and provider-payment decisions, and so do most public agencies. Thus care is restricted by the willingness of providers to deliver care at the payment level and of the patient to pay out of pocket. For this reason, many worry

that tightening budgets for public programs or cutbacks on employer payment levels for health plans shifts the financial risk to the individual and
implicitly rations according to the criteria of government or employers.

Proposals for voucher-style approaches (such as premium support proposals for Medicare and cash and counseling in Medicaid) or health savings accounts are said to respond to this concern by shifting greater
control of the financial resources to the beneficiaries of public programs
or private coverage. The aim in these approaches is to give beneficiaries
greater opportunity to shape the allocation of services according to their
own assessment of value and to remove it from government officials or
employers. But there are issues to consider in this approach. The community is at greater risk if the individual makes bad decisions (one reason
that HSAs are linked with catastrophic insurance). Moreover the resul-
tant balance of financial risk between the individual and the community
will depend on the way in which funds for the voucher or the savings
account are determined. The more that funding is indexed in some way to
the underlying cost of medical services, the less the risk is shifted to the
individual—and the less tightly health costs will be constrained. Still, as
discussed earlier, there remains under these approaches a tension between
community visions of value when public funds are involved and the individual's preferences. This tension is reflected in the degree to which benefit requirements are attached to the use of funds by the individual.

Rethinking the Medicare Social Contract

While many steps could be taken that would have some impact on the
explosive future growth in Medicare spending, it seems unlikely that dramatic savings can be achieved without redefining the Medicare promise.
Politically, revisiting that promise is no easy task. Americans would have
to agree on the nature of that promise as well as decide how sacrosanct
that promise is in the face of other goals and limited resources.

The actual Medicare promise is open to question. At its inception in
1965, the program's benefits reflected the objective of providing coverage
comparable to employment-based coverage at the time. If that objective
is held to remain the basis of the promise today, then it is reasonable to
modernize benefits, such as improving Medicare's catastrophic protection. It would also be in line with that view of the promise to alter

beneficiary costs to reflect the current trend toward greater cost-sharing in employment-based coverage. Alternatively, if the promise is to maintain the original approach to financial protection and the private-public balance of financial risk, it could seem reasonable to make significant adjustments today. For instance, the premium for Part B was originally set at 50 percent of costs. Today the beneficiary share is only 25 percent. Adjusting the premium percentage and the real value of deductibles to the original 1965 promise would mean substantial costs for seniors today and large savings to the program.

If it were possible to agree on what the promise is, would Americans be open to altering it to keep costs in check and free up resources for other social goals? Altering the promise would challenge deeply held values associated with the idea of social insurance. In particular, it would require Americans to alter the widespread view that Medicare is a sacrosanct social contract, a binding promise to deliver benefits based on an insurance agreement paid for not just with individual (subsidized) premiums and payroll taxes, but also collectively with general taxes. A step toward changing that view would be to correct the widespread misperception that promised benefits are financed entirely by payroll taxes and premiums and can be maintained by eliminating "waste" in Medicare itself and in other programs. To someone who holds this view, the solution to excessive costs is to improve efficiency, not renege on a promise. That person sees no trade-off between Medicare commitments and achieving other goals. To him or her, a proposal to reduce benefits or level of access to benefits is both unnecessary and unjust.

Thus if major changes are to be made in the benefits structure or financing of Medicare, Americans would have to think differently about the program and its underlying social values. That means redesigning the social insurance model. Of course, Medicare already departs significantly from the classic American social insurance model. Parts B and D are optional, premium-based insurance programs heavily subsidized by general revenue. Congress's decision to income test Part B premiums is a further departure.

Americans might be willing to modify the Medicare social contract. After all, Americans typically will forgo a portion of something they are entitled to if they accept the need for them to do so to address a higher need. Presenting more clearly in the budget process the scale of unfunded obligations and the growing role of general revenue in Medicare would help prepare the ground for a public discussion over the entitlement. That discussion would have to focus on the consequences for other national goals of honoring the letter of the Medicare promise, such as the crowding-out effect of the burgeoning general revenue commitment and the morality of passing on a huge financial burden to future generations.

Let us assume Americans were willing to contemplate a change in the Medicare social contract that would reduce the trajectory of costs and obligations in order to provide more resources for other goals and to reduce unfunded obligations. In what ways might the contract be reframed?

INCOME INSURANCE. One approach would be to turn Medicare into collective "income insurance" to enable retirees to afford adequate care if they lack sufficient income, rather than the traditional vision of social insurance. Income insurance would secure an individual's ability to afford health care during retirement. Risk insurance would replace today's program, which finances the delivery of medical benefits with little or no regard to income during retirement. Under this vision, today's income-related payroll taxes would become in effect a premium for collective insurance that pays for services only to the degree that an individual's retirement income falls below a certain level. In addition, upper-income retirees would pay an income-related premium for Part A services as well as Parts B and D or make payments in some other way. Individuals would in practice be paying income-adjusted premiums for a health program available to all retirees.

THE MEDICAID MODEL. Another approach would be to transform Medicare from a social insurance program into a more traditional income-based program. In effect Medicare would become a form of national Medicaid program for the elderly, with all benefits becoming income-related. Recent legislation to relate Part B premiums to income as well as unsuccessful proposals to make the drug benefit income-based assistance are consistent with this approach. Under this restructuring there would be a far weaker case for payroll tax financing, since the social insurance basis of Medicare would be replaced with a needs-based approach. To support this change, however, Americans would have to accept a crucial change in the nature of the Medicare promise. The program could no longer be interpreted as a promise to return dedicated contributions made during a person's working life—arguably a higher-order promise to return resources that somehow belong to the individual. Instead it would reflect a much more limited promise by the wider community to help the low-income elderly afford health care—a commitment that would have to compete on more equal terms with promises to other groups and for other purposes.

A third, hybrid approach would be to shrink the social insurance element of Medicare to the level of a very basic safety-net program, while encouraging or even mandating individual private savings and insurance to supplement the basic program. While keeping a smaller social insurance commitment in place, with its higher-order promise by the community, this approach would shift choice and responsibility for additional services to individuals. It would link supplementary benefits during retirement to the ability of the private savings and insurance vehicles to finance them, with the attendant risk to the individual, rather than to an open-ended commitment and shouldering of risk by the community.

Revising Expectations

If the proposals in this book are to be enacted, Americans will have to think differently about their expectations for health care, about the meaning of risk and mutual obligation, and about retirement. That will require a serious and honest conversation.

Americans will have to consider which health services should be a "membership right" for U.S. residents and which are marginal preferences. And given the aging of the baby boom generation, the idea of retirement must be at the center of that conversation. Rising costs associated with increased longevity, demographic shifts, and the health care expectations of a modern society are the principal drivers behind the country's health spending predicament.

A contemplation of the risks and promises related to retirement, and their implications for other groups and generations, is central to a discussion about retirement health costs. But so is a frank conversation about the very concept of retirement. As Barbara Butrica and others at the Urban Institute have pointed out, increasing life expectancy has changed expectations about retirement and fundamentally altered the economics of both private and public financing of retirement.[15] During the 1930s, when America began in earnest to create social insurance structures for retirement security, the typical worker could expect a retirement of just a few years—assuming he or she even reached retirement age. Today each new cohort of working Americans grows accustomed to the idea of enjoying an ever-larger proportion of its life in active retirement, financed in large part by someone else.

Americans so far have not been willing to accept significant limits in their health care. They also have yet to accept the proposition that the cost of generous health care during a predictably long retirement is unsustainable and cannot be shifted constantly to someone else. Anxiety about the uncertainties of health leads Americans to resist proposals to raise the Medicare eligibility age in line with increasing life expectancies (in contrast to Social Security where age was raised without much controversy). They are also resistant to the idea of curbing their ever-expanding health care expectations. And they are resistant to shouldering more of the predicable cost themselves while reserving social programs primarily for the needy and for truly unexpected developments. Until policymakers engage in a serious discussion with Americans about these issues and values, it will be very difficult to generate strong public support for the necessary steps to rein in health care costs.

Notes

1. Daniel Yankelovich, *Coming to Public Judgment: Making Democracy Work in a Complex World* (Syracuse University Press, 1991).

2. Indeed Malcolm Gladwell in his book *Blink: The Power of Thinking without Thinking* (New York: Little, Brown, 2005) refers to studies indicating that physicians who spend more time in conversation with their patients, and also engage in "active listening," are held in higher regard by patients and are far less likely to be sued. See Gladwell, pp. 39–43, referencing Wendy Levinson and others, "Physician-Patient Communication: The Relationship with Malpractice among Primary Care Physicians and Surgeons," *Journal of the American Medical Association* 277, no. 7 (1997), pp. 553–59.

3. For a discussion of efficiency and the particular challenges in achieving efficiency in health care, see Henry J. Aaron and William B. Schwartz, with Melissa Cox, *Can We Say No?: The Challenge of Rationing Health Care* (Brookings, 2005), pp. 93–107.

4. David M. Cutler, *Your Money or Your Life: Strong Medicine for America's Health Care System* (Oxford University Press, 2004), pp. 10–21.

5. If the transference of funds is seen as moving toward a Rawlsian vision of social justice through income equality, however, the funds would be interpreted as truly belonging to the recipient rather than the community, giving the community a much weaker claim to determining how the money is used.

6. For example, see Robert J. Blendon and John M. Benson, "Americans' Views on Health Policy: A Fifty-Year Historical Perspective," *Health Affairs* 20, no. 2 (March/April 2001): 33–46.

7. For example, Senator Joseph Lieberman (D-Conn.) introduced a comprehensive overhaul of the budget process in 2003 containing provisions requiring that unfunded liabilities be included in the budget process (S 1915 108th Cong., 1st sess., Honest Government Accounting Act of 2003).

8. For example, Rudolph G. Penner and C. Eugene Steuerle, "A Radical Proposal for Escaping the Budget Vise," *National Budget Issues* 3 (Washington: Urban Institute, June 2005) (urban.org/UploadedPDF/311192_NBI_3.pdf). The Medicare drug legislation of 2003 included a weak version of a trigger that would force consideration of a financing plan if general revenues were projected to rise above 45 percent of total Medicare costs—a proxy for the entitlement crowding out discretionary funds. Steuerle and Penner suggest a comprehensive trigger mechanism for retirement entitlements and for tax levels.

9. Robert J. Samuelson, "Affluence and Its Discontents," *Washington Post,* May 10, 2006, p. A25. See also Robert J. Samuelson, *The Good Life and Its Discontents* (New York: Crown, 1995).

10. C. Eugene Steuerle, "The Incredible Shrinking Budget for Working Families and Children," *National Budget Issues* 1 (Washington: Urban Institute, December 2003) (urban.org/UploadedPDF/310914_incredible_shrinking_budget.pdf).

11. For a proposal to combine national goals and policy parameters with wide state flexibility, see Henry J. Aaron and Stuart M. Butler, "How Federalism Could Spur Bipartisan Action on the Uninsured," *Health Affairs* web exclusive, March 31, 2004: W4-168–W4-178.

12. See Stuart M. Butler, "Private Sector Incentives and Ethical Health Care," in *Ethical Dimensions of Health Policy,* edited by Marion Danis, and Carolyn Clancy, and Larry R. Churchill (Oxford University Press, 2002), pp. 202–26.

13. For a description of the benefits board idea, see Stuart M. Butler, "Achieving Progress on Medicare," *Backgrounder* 1627 (Washington: Heritage Foundation, 2003) (www.heritage.org/Research/HealthCare/bg1627.cfm).

14. See Michael J. Garland, "Rationing in Public: Oregon's Priority-Setting Methodology," in *Rationing America's Medical Care: The Oregon Plan and Beyond,* edited by Martin A. Strosberg, Joshua M. Wiener, Robert Baker, and Alan Fein (Brookings, 1992), pp. 37–59.

15. Barbara A. Butrica, Karen E. Smith, and C. Eugene Steuerle, "Working for a Good Retirement," Retirement Project Discussion Paper 06-03 (Washington: Urban Institute, May 2006) (urban.org/UploadedPDF/311333_good_retirement.pdf).

Contributors

Joseph R. Antos
American Enterprise Institute

Stuart M. Butler
Heritage Foundation

Judith Feder
Georgetown Public Policy
   Institute

Paul B. Ginsburg
Center for Studying Health
   System Change

Susan D. Hosek
RAND Corporation

Donald W. Moran
The Moran Company

Alice M. Rivlin
Brookings Institution and
   Georgetown University

Louis F. Rossiter
College of William and Mary

Alan R. Weil
National Academy for State
   Health Policy

Gail R. Wilensky
Project HOPE

Index

Abortion, 10, 181
Aetna, 41, 162
Agency for Healthcare Research and Quality (AHRQ), 45, 51, 53, 56
AHCCCS. *See* Arizona Health Care Cost Containment System
AHLTA (Armed Forces Health Longitudinal Technology Application). *See* Health information technology—specific
AHRQ. *See* Agency for Healthcare Research and Quality
Alaska, 148
America. *See* North America; United States
Antos, Joseph, 13–28, 29–79, 126, 196, 197
Arizona Health Care Cost Containment System (AHCCCS), 117
Armed Forces Health Longitudinal Technology Application (AHLTA). *See* Health information technology—specific
Asch, Steven, 140

Baby-boom generation, 2, 23, 71, 88, 207
Balanced Budget Act of 1997, 83, 87, 89
Base Realignment and Closure process, 143
Beneficiaries: Medicaid and, 120–25; Medicare and, 84, 88, 91–92; reforms and, 6–7, 212; of VHA and MHS systems, 7, 143–45. *See also* Patients
Block grants: definition and use of, 113, 115; effects of, 114, 116, 207; Medicaid and, 6, 47t, 113–14; Medicare and, 98, 99
Boston (MA), 166. *See also* Massachusetts
Breaux, John (D-La.), 192n25
Breaux-Thomas model for Medicare, 183, 184
Budget issues: Clinton administration coverage strategy, 178; cost of health programs, 1–2, 4, 14–15, 16–17, 24, 142, 203; federal debt, 26; mandatory/entitlement spending, 20–22, 24, 25; Medicaid, 105–12, 115, 127,

204; Medicare, 184, 203, 204, 213–14; private health insurers, 8; reforms, 3, 9, 10, 184, 203–05; revenues, costs, and spending, 1–2, 9, 26; subsidies for worker insurance, 22; swap proposals, 114; VHA, 136
Burton, Alice, 121
Butler, Stuart, 10–11, 193–217
Butrica, Barbara, 215

California, 60, 68, 120, 123, 165
Canada, 17, 19, 211
Canadian National Health Service, 147
Capital Asset Realignment for Enhanced Services (CARES), 133
Capitation, 83, 116–18, 166
Care management programs, 86, 126
CARES. See Capital Asset Realignment for Enhanced Services
CARES Commission, 133
Case management programs, 56, 57
Cash and Counseling program, 63
CBO. See Congressional Budget Office
CDC. See Centers for Disease Control and Prevention
CEA. See Council of Economic Advisors
Census Bureau, 158, 160
Center for Evaluative Clinical Sciences (Dartmouth Medical School), 35
Centers for Disease Control and Prevention (CDC), 22, 60
Centers for Medicare and Medicaid Services (CMS): databases of, 126; disease management demonstrations and, 168; estimates of Medicaid spending, 107; fiscal gaming and, 115; gainsharing project of, 57; HIFA initiative of, 62–63; provider payments and, 91, 93; reforms and, 96, 163–64; research projects of, 51, 53, 64, 86
Centers of excellence, 157, 170n7
CHAMPUS (Civilian Health and Medical Program of the Uniformed Services; Department of Defense), 133–34
Children's issues, 107, 108, 111, 116, 175–76, 207. See also Medicaid

CIGNA, 41
Clinical trials, 36
Clinton, Bill, 113, 174
Clinton (Bill) administration, 9, 174–80
CMS. See Centers for Medicare and Medicaid Services
Cold War, 25, 133
Comparative Cost Adjustment Program, 62
Comparative effectiveness, 36, 54, 94, 95, 97, 188, 189
Congressional Budget Office (CBO), 14, 69, 89, 138, 179
Connecticut, 123
Conservatives, 183–84. See also Political issues
Cost sharing: bidding and, 49; Clinton administration reforms and, 178; in emergency departments, 59; employer-provided and private payer plans and, 148, 154, 159, 162, 163, 212–13; HIFA initiative of 2001, 62–63; MCAA and, 182; Medicaid and, 107, 110, 122, 127, 163; Medicare and, 87, 89–90, 91, 100, 101, 107, 163; physicians and, 164; prescription drugs and, 161; proposals and reforms for, 7, 65, 148; VA and DoD and, 132, 133, 134, 138–39, 144
Cost shifting. See Economic issues
Coughlin, Teresa A., 116
Council of Economic Advisors (CEA), 15
Cutler, David, 196

Dartmouth Medical School. See Center for Evaluative Clinical Sciences
Defense, Department of (DoD): EMR system in, 7–8, 141, 145, 146; health care spending and, 132; health programs of, 22, 44, 132, 133; medical personnel requirement of, 142; outsourcing MHS care, 142–43; prescription drugs and, 50; quality of care and, 141; spending of, 25. See also Military Health System; TRICARE
Deficit Reduction Act (2005), 63, 120

Defined benefit plans, 120–21, 183,
    204, 206
Defined contribution plans, 6–7, 120,
    121, 183
Delivery of health care. *See* Health care
Democratic Party, 113–14, 184. *See also*
    Political issues
Demographic factors: age, 2, 17, 20;
    effects of, 20, 23; infant mortality,
    17; life expectancy, 2, 17, 23, 60, 90,
    122–23, 215–16
Diagnosis-related groups (DRGs),
    85–86, 87, 96, 164. *See also*
    Hospitals
Direct purchase models, 120–21
Disabilities and the disabled: Medicaid
    and, 107, 108, 116, 117, 127;
    Medicare and, 97, 175; veterans,
    133, 136
Disease management programs: defini-
    tion and elements of, 56–57, 167;
    effectiveness and wellness and,
    167–69; insurance and, 163;
    Medicaid and, 56, 107, 110,
    118–19; Medicare and, 157–58;
    reforms and, 6
Diseases and disorders: asthma, 118,
    163; cardiovascular disease, 59, 86,
    118, 163; catastrophic injury, 142;
    chronic diseases, 59, 86, 118, 127,
    168; combat injuries, 148; develop-
    mental disorders, 107; diabetes, 59,
    86, 118, 163; HIV/AIDS, 107, 126;
    mental illness, 107; neurological dis-
    orders, 107; obesity, 59–60; post-
    traumatic stress disorder, 142; spinal
    cord injuries, 107; traumatic brain
    injuries, 126
DoD. *See* Defense, Department of
DRGs. *See* Diagnosis-related groups;
    Hospitals
Drug Price Competition and Patent
    Term Restoration Act. *See* Hatch-
    Waxman Act
Drugs. *See* Prescription drugs

Economic issues: competition, 30, 40,
    47t, 61–65, 178–79; consumerism,

61–65, 162; cost containment,
    185–90; cost-effectiveness, 54, 60,
    126, 139–41; cost shifting and redis-
    tribution, 112, 114, 156, 177–79;
    crisis in health care finance, 185; dis-
    ease management, 57; economic
    cycles, 111, 158; efficiency in health
    care, 195–96; employment-based
    insurance, 38; fiscal gaming, 115–16,
    205; gross domestic product (GDP),
    23, 24, 25, 70–71, 201; growth fac-
    tors, 114; health care costs, 9, 20,
    177, 199–202; income levels, 34–35,
    60, 90, 110, 111, 112, 124; interest
    rates, 26; market-based reforms, 3, 4,
    39–41, 43, 210; National Health
    Expenditures (NHE), 24, 106; per-
    ceptions of value and efficiency,
    196–97; personal discretionary
    income, 20; regulatory-based
    reforms, 3, 4; risk and risk shifting,
    63, 121, 205–09; supply and
    demand, 32, 36, 40; third-party pay-
    ments, 20. *See also* Budget issues;
    Cost sharing; Employment issues;
    Health care costs and spending;
    Subsidies; Taxes and tax issues
EDs (emergency departments). *See*
    Hospitals
Educational issues, 22, 98
Elderly and seniors, 1–2, 5, 21, 23, 33.
    See also Demographic factors;
    Medicaid; Medicare
Election of 2000, 180
Electronic medical records (EMR). *See*
    Health information technology—
    specific
Emergency departments (EDs). *See*
    Hospitals
Emergency Medical Treatment and
    Active Labor Act (EMTALA; 1986),
    58
Employment issues: Clinton administra-
    tion coverage strategy, 178; cost of
    employer-sponsored coverage, 177;
    disease management programs, 168;
    employee and retiree health costs, 25,
    124, 143, 154; health assessments,

168; health behaviors, 122, 187, 197; health savings accounts, 64; managed care, 33, 56, 158; Medicaid, 124, 125, 154, 176; private health insurance, 158–59, 163, 174–75, 197; public health insurance, 175; quality of care, 157; subsidies and tax exclusions for health insurance, 4, 8, 32, 34, 38, 44–45, 62, 65, 153, 158, 175, 178, 197–98, 200; VHA and MHS users, 144–45

EMR (Electronic medical records). *See* Health information technology—specific

EMTALA. *See* Emergency Medical Treatment and Active Labor Act

End of life. *See* Health care

Entitlement programs, 20–22, 25, 34, 202, 203–05, 206–07. *See also* Medicaid; Medicare; Social Security; Subsidies

Ethics issues. *See* Moral, ethics, and social issues

EU. *See* European Union

Europe, 17, 18, 19, 133. *See also individual countries*

European Union (EU), 19. *See also individual countries*

Evidence-based medicine, 31, 32

Exercise, 59–60

Fast food, 60

FDA. *See* Food and Drug Administration

Federal Employees Health Benefits Program (FEHBP), 40, 51, 61, 64, 92, 121

Federal government. *See* Government, federal

Federal Supply Schedule, 50, 140, 147

Federal Trade Commission (FTC), 4, 45, 67

Feder, Judith, 9–10, 173–92

Fee-for-service programs: effects of, 36, 37, 45, 47; Medicaid and, 56, 117; Medicare and, 83–84; seniors and, 83

FEHBP. *See* Federal Employees Health Benefits Program

Financial incentives. *See* Incentives

Florida, 63, 120

Food and Drug Administration (FDA): approval of biologics, 68; approval of prescription drugs, 65–68; Critical Path Initiative of, 66–67; mission and role of, 4, 78n82; regulation of health sector and, 45

FTC. *See* Federal Trade Commission

GAO. *See* Government Accountability Office

Ginsburg, Paul, 8–9, 153–71, 197

Goldberg, Mathew, 140

Government Accountability Office (GAO), 115, 124

Government, federal: block grants and, 113; comparative effectiveness center and, 94; health data development and research by, 53–54, 55, 162–63, 189–90; health programs of, 44–45; health spending by, 1–2, 13–25, 106, 168; leadership in reforms, 4–5, 39, 44–45, 95–97; Medicaid and, 21, 105, 107, 108, 109–10, 113–14; performance measurement systems and, 6; premium support and, 61; prescription drugs and, 50; reform options for federal health programs, 46–47; risk reduction and, 207–08; role in healthcare, 30; unsustainability of health care costs and, 25–26. *See also* Agency for Healthcare Research and Quality; Federal Employees Health Benefits Program; Medicaid; Medicare

Government, state: block grants to, 6, 113; fiscal gaming by, 6, 115; health spending by, 106; Medicaid and state health programs and, 6, 21–22, 25, 62–63, 105, 107, 108, 109–10, 111, 113–20, 123, 125; risk reduction and, 207–08; social and welfare benefits of, 110. *See also* Medicaid

Hadley, Jack, 107

Hatch-Waxman Act (Drug Price Competition and Patent Term Restoration Act; *1984*), 68

Hawaii, 35
Health and Human Services, Department of (HHS), 51
Health care: as an art, 35; clinical guidelines and management, 55–57; community standards for acceptable care, 70, 120; cost-effectiveness of, 54; cost sharing and, 163; defensive medicine, 69; delivery of, 2, 17, 46, 55–61, 116–20; efficiency and effectiveness of, 17, 20, 35–38, 39, 195–200; end-of-life care, 58, 84; expectations for, 215–16; fairness and equity of, 195–200, 205, 208–10; improvements in, 1, 6, 15, 16–17, 19–20; information regarding, 36, 40, 46, 94; patient outcomes and, 36, 196; rationing of, 54, 179, 187, 209–12; risk and, 205–09; quality of care, 8–9, 31, 41, 51, 55–56, 69, 85–86, 120, 159; universal health care, 3, 43. See also Employment issues; Insurance and insurers; Reforms; Moral, ethics, and social issues
Health care costs and spending: amount of, 13, 35, 41; bundling and, 40–41, 57; control/containment of, 9, 10, 41, 42–43, 70–71, 185–90; effects of changes, 200–202; efficiency of, 35, 194, 200–201; end-of-life care and, 58, 84; government spending, 20–26, 34–35, 154, 174; health promotion and disease prevention and, 59–61; increases in, 1–2, 3, 5, 9, 13–15, 17–20, 22–25, 176–77; malpractice insurance and, 68; public support for slowing growth, 193–216; role of private payers in, 153–69; setting prices or payment rates, 45–50; strategies for slowing the growth of, 3–6, 16–17, 31–32, 47t, 174, 177, 178; third-party payments and, 33; unsustainability of, 25–26, 32, 70–71, 216. See also Reforms; Subsidies; Taxes and tax issues
Healthcare Quality Initiatives Review Panel (Department of Defense), 141

Health care systems: administration and administrative costs of, 18; complexity, fragmentation, and interconnectedness of, 1, 3, 18, 32; efficiency of, 36. See also Military Health System; Private health plans and insurers; Public health plans and insurers; Reforms; Veterans Health Administration; individual programs
Health information technology: costs of, 52; current developments, 4–5, 31, 50–55; data collection and, 52–53, 126; patient privacy and, 52; pay-for-performance and, 167; proposals for, 4; treatment options and, 37; VHA and MHS innovations, 7–8
Health information technology— specific: Armed Forces Health Longitudinal Technology Application (AHLTA), 7–8, 146; electronic medical records (EMR), 7, 51, 52, 66, 146; Veterans Health Information System and Technology Architecture (VistA), 7, 51, 145–46
Health Insurance Association of America, 180
Health Insurance Flexibility and Accountability (HIFA; 2001), 6–63
Health Insurance Plans, 160
Health maintenance organizations (HMOs), 56, 83, 116, 134, 144. See also Managed care
Health savings accounts (HSAs). See Insurance and insurers
HHS. See Health and Human Services, Department of
HIFA. See Health Insurance Flexibility and Accountability
High-performance networks. See Physicians
HMOs. See Health maintenance organizations
Holahan, John, 107
Home-based care, 122
Hosek, Susan, 7–8, 131–51
Hospice, 58

Hospitals: bundled payments for, 87; costs of, 156; cost sharing and, 163; diagnosis-related group reimbursement, 85–86, 87; effects of supply on usage, 36; efficiency of, 48, 162; gainsharing by, 57, 86; incentives for, 85; Medicaid and, 107; Medicare Part A (Hospital Insurance program) and, 82; payment rates for, 156–57, 164–65; prospective payment systems for, 47–48, 188–89; quality of care, 85–86, 159, 165; tiered hospital networks, 161; use of emergency services, 39, 58

HSAs (health savings accounts). *See* Insurance and insurers

IHS. *See* Indian Health Service

Incentives: clinical guidelines and, 55–56; effects of, 6–7, 34, 61; for hospitals, 57, 86; in Medicaid, 109–10, 113–16, 119–20, 121–22, 123–24; in Medicare, 84–85, 91–94, 95; negative and reverse incentives, 93, 169, 187–88; for patients, 121–22, 123–24, 159–64, 169, 188; for pharmaceutical manufacturers, 188; for physicians, 57, 86, 166; for promotion of higher quality of care, 165–67; for providers, 85, 94–95, 97, 147–48, 188; reforms and, 38, 47–48, 113–16, 194–95; use of, 8, 10–11, 57. *See also* Subsidies

Incentives—specific: bundling, 84, 85; cost sharing, 91; fee-for-service payments, 57, 84–85; gainsharing, 57, 86; high-performance networks, 8–9; partnership programs, 123–24; patient agreements, 69, 121–22, 159–64; pay-for-performance, 9, 43, 48–49, 57, 92–93, 94–95, 119–20, 166; premium support, 61; prospective payment systems, 47–48, 84; swaps, 114. *See also* Block grants

Indiana, 123

Indian Health Service (IHS), 51, 148, 149n1

Information. *See* Health care; Health information technology

Institute of Medicine (IOM), 93–94, 147

Insurance and insurers: Clinton administration coverage strategy, 177–80; cost containment and, 187–89; coverage and coverage expansion, 42, 176–77; data development by, 53, 162–63; health information technology use by, 51; medical necessity standards and, 54–55; private payer role in health spending, 153–69; prospective payment plans and, 188–89; reimbursement and payment, 54–55, 164; treatment versus prevention and, 37–38; under-65 population and, 83; universal coverage and, 174, 175. *See also* Employment issues; Managed care; Medicaid; Medicare; Military Health System; Private health plans and insurers; TRICARE; Veterans Health Administration

Insurance and insurers—premiums and cost sharing: co-payments and deductibles, 33, 40, 41, 64, 159, 188; premium assistance, 62–63, 124; premiums and cost of, 34, 38; premium caps, 179; premium support, 61–62, 92; stop-loss provisions, 82; subsidies for, 154; tax factors and, 34–35, 64–65, 79n105, 153–54

Insurance and insurers—specific: health savings and other accounts, 40, 64, 77n76, 85, 160; income insurance, 11, 214; long-term and end-of-life care insurance, 7, 58, 112, 117, 122–24, 125; malpractice insurance, 68; Medigap and Medicare supplementary insurance, 82, 91; military insurance, 133–34; reinsurance, 125; risk and risk insurance, 206, 214; tiered coinsurance, 91

Integrated Healthcare Association, 165

IOM. *See* Institute of Medicine

"It's the economy, Stupid" (Clinton administration), 174

Japan, 17, 19

Joint Committee on Taxation, 65

Kerr, Eva A., 140
King County (WA), 168. *See also* Seattle

Leapfrog Group, 43, 159
Long-term care, 7, 117, 122–24, 125
Louisiana, 107

Maine, 107
Malpractice and malpractice reform, 4, 31, 32, 68–69
Managed care and managed care plans: capitation arrangements and, 116–18; costs and cost containment and, 83, 187; disease management and, 118; effects of, 155; efficiency of, 47; high-performance networks and, 162; Medicaid and, 111–12, 116–18, 155; Medicare and, 47, 155, 191n21; popularity of, 56, 187; prescription drugs and, 182; prospective payment plans and, 188–89; quality of care and, 8; referrals in, 33; reforms and, 6; VHA and, 135–36. *See also* Health maintenance organizations
Massachusetts, 154, 169n2. *See also* Boston
MCAA. *See* Medicare Catastrophic Coverage Act
Medicaid: background of, 174; as a data source, 52–53, 119; demand for, 122–25; effects on U.S. health care system of, 44; efficiency of, 110, 111, 112, 114–15; growth of, 6, 14, 107, 175–76; health care delivery and, 116–20; health information technology and, 126; new technologies and, 155; role of, 6, 13–14, 27n14, 32, 33–34, 38, 107–08, 112, 122, 128, 175, 190n3; seniors and, 108, 117; smoking and, 60. *See also* Disabilities and the disabled
Medicaid—economic issues: costs and spending, 2, 4, 6, 7, 14, 20, 21–22, 42, 54, 70, 105, 107, 111–28; cost sharing, 110, 122, 127; per capita cap, 113–14; place in budgets and the health system, 105–12; fiscal gaming, 115–16; premium assistance

programs, 124; projections of spending for, 22–24, 29, 107; providers and provider payment rates, 107, 111–12, 119–20; reforms, 4, 6–7, 47t, 62–63, 112–28, 203–05, 209
Medicaid—plan characteristics: benefits, 108, 109, 114, 120, 122; as a defined benefit plan, 120, 121, 202; as a defined contribution plan, 120, 121; disease and care management programs, 118–19, 126; eligibility, 7, 110, 111, 112, 125, 175–76, 190n6; emergency room services, 59; end-of-life care, 58; enrollees and enrollment, 107, 108, 127, 163; fee-for-service payments, 118; home-based care, 122; links with Medicare, 57, 126–27; long-term care, 122–25; managed care, 56, 110, 116–18; pay-for-performance system, 119–20, 126; personal care services, 63; policy models, 120–22; prescription drug program, 50; structural uniqueness, 109–12
Medical equipment, 18, 49, 95–96
Medical Injury Compensation Reform Act (MICRA; *1975*; CA), 68
Medicare: background of, 81–88, 174; as a data source, 52–53, 119; effects of, 44, 157; efficiency of, 91–92; growth of, 14, 87–88; health information technology and, 51; patient outcomes and, 36; public attitudes and views toward, 11, 212–15; quality of care and, 85, 157; role and objectives of, 13, 32, 72n1, 81–82, 88, 175, 212–15; seniors and elderly and, 33, 56, 58, 82, 84, 92, 168, 175, 209. *See also* Hospice; Nursing home care
Medicare—economic issues: benefits and benefit limits, 89–91, 164; bidding and, 49–50, 95; bundling and, 57, 84, 92; cost containment and, 187–88; costs and spending, 2, 4, 5–6, 14, 20, 21, 35–36, 42, 47–50, 62, 83–85, 87–101, 176, 212–13; cost sharing and, 90, 91, 163, 212–13; physician and provider

compensation and, 70–71, 84–85,
187–88; premiums for, 61–62, 71,
92, 97, 213; projections of spending
for, 22–24, 29, 163; reforms and, 4,
5–6, 11, 47–48, 61–62, 88–101, 176,
182–85, 203–05, 209, 212–15; reimbursement methods, 164, 165;
resource use and, 36; subsidies and,
8, 62
Medicare—program characteristics: case
management programs, 57; as a
defined benefit plan, 183, 202; as a
defined contribution plan, 120, 183;
disease management programs and,
57, 168; eligibility age, 90, 103n18;
end-of-life care and, 58; fee-for-service payments, 36, 47, 84–85, 86,
97; health savings accounts and, 64;
Health Support pilot program, 86;
links with Medicaid and, 57,
126–27, 190n3; managed care and,
47, 155, 191n21; nursing home care,
108, 111, 122–23; Parts/components
of, 82, 90–91, 120, 213; pay-for-performance system and, 48–49, 92–94,
96–97, 157, 166; prescription drug
benefit, 20, 49–50, 62, 82–83, 154,
181–85, 191n21; prospective payment system and, 47–48, 84
Medicare Advantage (Part C) plans:
choice of health plans under, 61–62,
77n79, 82, 154; managed care and,
47; patient financial incentives and,
164; patient outcomes and, 140; pay-
for-performance plans and, 48, 96;
price competition and, 62; special
needs and, 127
Medicare Catastrophic Coverage Act
(MCAA; 1988), 182
Medicare Modernization Act (MMA;
2003), 10, 62, 83, 90, 96, 126–27,
181-85
Medicare Payment Advisory Commission (MedPAC), 87, 88–89, 91, 156
Medicare Trustees, 203
MedPAC. See Medicare Payment Advisory Commission
Mental health and illness, 107, 117
MHS. See Military Health System

Miami (FL), 35
MICRA. See Medical Injury Compensation Reform Act
Military Health System (MHS): benefits
of, 143–45; coordination of care,
145–46; cost-effectiveness of care,
139–41, 143; cost sharing and, 132,
138–39; coverage of, 7, 142; evolution of health care in, 132–33,
145–46; expansion and choices of
military health care, 133–34, 135f,
142; funding and spending by, 131,
142; medical personnel requirements,
142; options for provision of health
care by, 141–45; performance incentives of, 147–48; prescription drug
plan of, 140, 147; quality of care in,
140, 143, 147; reforms and, 7–8;
trends in users and budgets of, 137.
See also Defense, Department of
Military treatment facilities (MTFs),
133–34, 141, 142–43
Milligan, Charles, 121
Minneapolis (MN), 35
Mississippi, 107
Missouri, 107
Moral, ethics, and social issues: cost-
effectiveness, 54; in health care, 32,
42, 70, 71, 187, 196–202; of insurance, 34; limiting growth of spending, 200–202; moral hazard, 33, 34,
40; private versus social perceptions
of value and efficiency, 196–200;
rationing, 210; social promises,
202–16
Moran, Donald W., 9–10, 173–92
MTFs. See Military treatment facilities

National Academy for State Health Pol-
icy, 116
National Bipartisan Commission on the
Future of Medicare, 183
National Committee for Quality Assur-
ance (NCQA), 96
National eligibility standards, 125
National Health Expenditures (NHE),
24, 106
National Institutes of Health (NIH), 22,
45

National Quality Forum (NQF), 96
NCQA. *See* National Committee for Quality Assurance
Neurological disorders, 107
New Jersey, 35–36
New York, 35, 120, 123
NHE. *See* National Health Expenditures
NIH. *See* National Institutes of Health
Nixon, Richard M., 176
North America, 17. *See also individual countries and states*
NQF. *See* National Quality Forum
Nugent, Gary N., 140
Nurses, 18, 57
Nursing home care. *See* Medicare— program characteristics

OECD. *See* Organization for Economic Cooperation and Development
Office of Generic Drug Approval (Food and Drug Administration), 67
Office of Management and Budget (OMB), 109, 153
Ohio, 35–36
OMB. *See* Office of Management and Budget
Oregon, 35
Oregon Health Plan, 54, 70, 211
Organization for Economic Cooperation and Development (OECD), 17, 18–19

PACE. *See* Program of All-Inclusive Care for the Elderly
Partnership programs, 123
Patients: costs and prices of services and, 40–41; cost sharing and, 163, 164; disease management and, 118; efficient use of health care by, 91–92; failure to adhere to treatment regimen, 60–61; high-cost patients, 41; incentives for, 121–22, 123–24, 159–64; information and knowledge of, 37, 40, 41, 92, 120; malpractice and, 68, 69; market reform strategies and, 39–40; role in their own health care, 56, 127, 159. *See also* Beneficiaries

Pay-for-performance (P4P): effects on spending, 166–67; formulas for, 96; as an incentive for higher quality care, 9, 43, 48–49, 85, 92–93, 94, 165, 166–67; questions and controversies regarding, 48; reforms and, 4, 6, 31, 32, 96–97, 126; standards of performance and, 57, 120. *See also* Medicaid; Medicare
Payment-for-results model, 94
P4P. *See* Pay-for-performance
PDPs. *See* Prescription drug plans
Pennsylvania, 107, 120
Performance Measurement: Accelerating Improvement (report, Institute of Medicine), 93
Performance measurement system, 6, 93
Pharmaceutical industry, 182, 183. *See also* Prescription drugs
Pharmaceutical Research and Manufacturers of America (PhRMA), 182–84
PHS. *See* Public Health Service
Physicians: clinical guidelines and, 55; compensation, fees, and payment rates for, 18, 70–71, 89, 92, 157, 164; defensive medicine and, 69; efficiency of, 162; gainsharing by, 57, 86; gatekeepers and referrals, 33; high-performance networks of, 9, 161–62; information use and management by, 37, 51, 52; malpractice insurance of, 68; Medicare Part B (Supplementary Medical Insurance program) and, 82, 84–85, 86–87, 89, 90, 92, 166, 199; practice size and, 167; private and public patients of, 156; quality of care of, 86, 92, 162, 165–66; in the U.S., 18. *See also* Providers
Pitney Bowes, 163
Point of Service (POS) programs, 83
Policies and policy options: Medicare, 70–71; policy decisionmaking, 194; proposals for, 4, 10–11; setting prices or payment rates, 45–50; spending for health care and, 15, 71, 200–202. *See also* Reforms

Political issues: Clinton health reform plan, 174, 177, 179–80; competitive pricing, 62; fiscal gaming, 115; health care costs and spending, 20–21, 173–90, 193–216; health care reforms, 9–10, 30, 39, 65, 71, 148, 173–90, 215–16; Medicaid, 111, 125, 163, 175; Medicare, 5, 70–71, 81, 91, 96, 97, 163, 175; Medicare Modernization Act, 181–85; polarization and partisanship, 9–10, 180–81, 183–85; prescription drug plans, 144, 182–85; public support for health care reform, 10–11, 177; seniors/elderly, 5, 21, 23, 175

POS. *See* Point of Service programs

PPOs. *See* Preferred provider organizations

PPS. *See* Prospective payment system

Preferred provider organizations and options (PPOs), 56, 83, 134

Premier Inc., 85–86

Premium assistance programs, 124

Prepaid health plans, 116

Prescription drug plans (PDPs), 49–50. *See also* Medicaid; Medicare; Military Health System; Veterans Health Administration

Prescription drugs: analgesics, 65; approval process for, 65–68; biologics, 67–68, 160; branded drugs, 67; costs and prices of, 18, 50, 67, 68, 147, 182; cost sharing and, 161, 163; generic drugs, 8–9, 67, 68, 160, 161, 163; private payer benefits, 159–60; reforms for, 66, 67; tiered structure of, 159–60, 161, 188. *See also* Pharmaceutical industry

Prevention: health care costs and spending and, 60; insurers and, 37–38; mammography, 36; medical screening, 60; role in reform, 31–32; smoking cessation programs, 60; uninsured population and, 38–39; use of services, 36; vaccinations, 36, 60

Primary care case management programs, 56

Private health plans and insurers: actuarial value of, 159; in Boston, 166; consumer-driven health plans, 160; costs and spending of, 9, 85, 87–88, 187; coverage and enrollment of, 7, 160; data development by, 163; disease management and, 168; links with public insurers, 8, 169; for long-term care, 123; Medicare and, 83; premiums, 158, 187; prescription drug benefits, 159–60; private payer initiatives, 158–69; quality of care and, 93, 165–66; reforms and, 3, 6; role of, 33; subsidies for, 34; VistA and, 7. *See also* Employment issues; Health care systems; Insurance and insurers

Program of All-Inclusive Care for the Elderly (PACE), 117, 118

Prospective payment system (PPS), 47–48, 74n25, 84, 188–89

Providers: business aspects of medical practice, 37; case management and, 56; centers of excellence, 157; as a common delivery system, 8, 17, 154–55; efficiency of, 162; information use by, 36–37, 56; Medicaid and, 107, 11–12, 154–55; Medicare and, 84–85, 89, 91, 92, 154–55; networks, 170n5; patient incentives and choice and, 161; quality of care and, 8, 41, 92, 157; reforms and, 6, 40, 97; reimbursement methods, 164–65; TRICARE and, 154–55. *See also* Fee-for-service payment; High-performance networks; Incentives; Physicians

Public health plans and insurers: cost of health care and, 9, 187, 201–02; coverage of, 175–76; establishment of, 175; high-performance networks and, 162; links with private insurers, 8; reforms and, 17; value in, 199–200. *See also* Medicaid; Medicare; Military Health System; TRICARE; Veterans Health Administration

Public Health Service (PHS), 5

Public policies. *See* Policies and policy options

Quality Enhancement Research Initiative (QUERI; Veterans Health Administration), 147

RAND, 110
Rationing, 209–12
RBRVS. *See* Resource-Based Relative Value Scale
Reagan, Ronald, 114
Reagan (Ronald) administration, 91
Referrals. *See* Managed care
Reforms: approaches to, 3, 30–32; barriers to, 9; Benefits Board, 211; Clinton reform plan, 174–80; competitive reforms, 30; comprehensive reforms, 30–39; cost controls/containment, 9, 10, 41, 42–43, 185–90; goals and objectives of, 2, 3–4, 39; market-based reforms, 3, 4, 39–41, 43; moral and social factors, 11; need for, 25–26, 30–39; options for federal health activities, 46–47; political factors, 9–10, 30, 39, 173–90, 193–216; prescription drugs and, 182–85; previous attempts at, 3, 9; pricing reforms, 47–48; private payer role in reforms, 153–69; proposals for, 4, 5–11, 98–101; public support for, 173; regulatory-based reforms, 3, 4, 42–43, 70; strategies for, 39–43; universal system reforms, 30; VHA and MHS and, 131–32. *See also* Health information technology; Medicaid; Medicare; Policies and policy options
Republican Party, 183–84. *See also* Political issues
Research: approval process for prescription drugs, 65–68; on coordination of care, 146–47; on costs and cost-effectiveness of care, 140–41, 143, 189–90; data development, 52–53, 66; on disease management, 157, 167–68; on effective treatment, 36–37; on Medicaid managed care,

116–17; on Medicare P4P, 166; on quality of care, 85–86, 140, 141, 147; on health system improvements, 45, 96; RAND health insurance experiment, 110; research outcomes and effectiveness, 53–55; Social Security Act waivers and, 109; state governments and Medicaid and, 110. *See also* Health information technology
Research—specific methods: clinical trials, 36, 53, 54, 66, 67, 186; comparative effectiveness studies, 36, 54; Critical Path Initiative (FDA), 66–67; demonstration projects, 49, 51, 57, 85–87, 96, 116–17, 146, 157, 166, 168; head-to-head trials, 66; pilot projects, 85–86
Resource-Based Relative Value Scale (RBRVS), 96
Retirement: of baby boomers, 2, 20, 23, 88; income insurance and, 11, 214, 215–16; Medicare and, 209; planning for, 204
Rivlin, Alice M., 13–28, 29–79, 126, 196, 197
Rossiter, Louis F., 6–7, 105–30

St. Paul Companies, 68
Samuelson, Robert, 206
SCHIP. *See* State Children's Health Insurance Program
Seattle (WA), 162. *See also* King County
Selim, Alfredo J., 140
Seniors. *See* Elderly and seniors; Medicaid; Medicare
SGR. *See* Sustainable growth rate
Single-payer systems, 3
Smoking, 60
Social issues. *See* Moral, ethics, and social issues
Social Security: cost of, 14; Disability Insurance program, 72n1; effects on future budgets, 13; eligibility age for, 90; Medicare deductions and, 182; projections of spending for, 22–23; taxes and, 82
Social Security Act (*1935*), 109
Special needs patients and plans, 126–27

Spending. *See* Health care costs and spending; *individual programs*

State Children's Health Insurance Program (SCHIP), 32–33, 44, 62–63, 71–72, 176

State government. *See* Government, state

Stem cell research, 10, 181

Steuerle, Eugene, 207

Subsidies: caps on, 65; effects of, 33–34; for insurance, 4, 8, 22, 154; Medicaid and, 154; Medicare and, 62, 90–91, 154; partnership programs, 123; reforms and, 194–95. *See also* Incentives; Taxes and tax issues

Sustainable growth rate (SGR), 70–71, 85

Switzerland, 17

Taxes and tax issues: federal entitlements and, 14; federal health programs and, 1–2; health savings accounts, 64, 160; insurance, 34–35, 64–65, 79n105, 153–54; Medicaid-related tax credits, 125; reforms and, 44–45, 214; Social Security wage tax, 82; subsidies and tax exclusions for health insurance, 4, 8, 32, 34–35, 38, 44–45, 62, 64–65, 72n5, 77n76, 153, 158, 175, 178, 197–98, 200; tax increases, 26

Tennessee, 107

Texas, 120

Third-party plans and payments, 20, 32–35, 40, 42

Thomas, Bill (R-CA), 192n25. *See also* Breaux-Thomas model for Medicare

Tiering: coinsurance, 91; prescription drugs, 159–60, 161, 188; principle of, 208

Tort reforms, 68–69

Toyota Production System, 162

TRICARE program (Department of Defense): background and programs of, 133–34, 136; coordination of care and, 146, 147; costs of, 71–72, 137, 140–41; cost sharing in, 138, 144; enrollment in, 142; information technology and, 51; premiums for, 143–44; prescription drug plan of, 144; reforms and, 44; role of, 170n3

Uninsured population: access to health care of, 38–39; changes to federal-state partnership for, 125; Clinton administration coverage strategy and, 177; cost of health care and, 9, 38–39, 177; cost of insurance and, 177; Medicaid and Medicare and, 29, 174, 176; number of uninsureds, 16, 30, 33, 38, 73n12, 175, 177; problems of, 38–39, 174; use of emergency departments, 58

United Kingdom, 17, 211

United States: health care system in, 1–2, 5, 15–16, 17–18, 19, 32, 43, 56; health habits in, 59; national health expenditures in, 106; public views of reforms, 203, 213; quality of life in, 1; sense of fairness in, 209; spending on health care in, 15–17, 29, 59; views of Medicare in, 213; views of risk in, 205–09. *See also individual states*

Utah, 35

Veterans Affairs, Department of (VA): health care spending and, 132; health programs of, 132; prescription drugs and, 50; quality of care and, 155; reforms in, 4–5

Veterans Health Administration (VHA): benefits of, 143–45; coordination of care, 146–47; cost-effectiveness of care, 139–41, 143; cost sharing and, 132, 138–39; coverage of, 7, 134; eligibility and enrollment in, 135, 136–39, 141–42, 143; evolution of health care in, 132–33, 145–46; expansion of veterans' health care, 134–36; funding and spending of, 131, 136–39, 142; health information technology use by, 51; managed care and, 135–36; options for provision of health care by, 141–45; performance incentives of, 147–48; premiums for, 143; prescription drug plan of, 140, 144, 147; quality of care of, 140, 143, 147; reforms and, 4–5, 7–8, 44, 71–72

Veterans' Health Care Eligibility Reform
    Act of *1996*, 135
Veterans Health Information System and
    Technology Architecture (VistA). *See*
    Health information technology—
    specific
VHA. *See* Veterans Health
    Administration
Vioxx, 65
Virginia Mason Medical Center
    (VMMC; Seattle), 162
VistA (Veterans Health Information Sys-
    tem and Technology Architecture).
    See Health information technology—
    specific

VMMC. *See* Virginia Mason Medical
    Center
Vouchers, 121, 212

Weil, Alan, 6–7, 105–30
Wennberg, Jack, 35
West Virginia, 60–61, 121
Wilensky, Gail, 5–6, 81–103, 197
Woodcock, Cynthia, 121
World War II, 133, 135
Wyoming, 107

Yankelovich, Daniel, 193–94

Zuckerman, Stephen, 116